Diary

Also by Richard Selzer

Richard Selzer

Diary

Yale

UNIVERSITY PRESS

 New Haven and London

Yale University Press books may be purchased in quantity for educational, business, or promotional use. For information, please e-mail sales.press@yale.edu (U.S. office) or sales@yaleup.co.uk (U.K. office).

Designed by Sonia Shannon

Set in Fournier type by Keystone Typesetting, Inc.

Printed in the United States of America by Thomson-Shore, Inc.

Library of Congress Cataloging-in-Publication Data

Selzer, Richard, 1928–

Diary / Richard Selzer.

   p. cm.

ISBN 978-0-300-12461-3 (alk. paper)

1. Selzer, Richard, 1928– 2. Authors, American—20th century—Biography. I. Title.

PS3569.E585Z46 2010

813'.54—dc22

[B]   2010007988

A catalogue record for this book is available from the British Library.

This paper meets the requirements of ANSI/NISO Z39.48-1992 (Permanence of Paper).

10 9 8 7 6 5 4 3 2 1

To Janet and her three daughters-in-law:
Regine (Jon), Rossi (Larry), and Donna (Gretchen)

Tell all the truth but tell it slant.
—Emily Dickinson

Contents

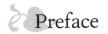# Preface

TO KEEP A DIARY is an act of egotism, an announcement that your life is a cabinet of curiosities interesting enough and amusing enough to warrant the attention of readers. Unlike the painter Delacroix (my idea of a great diarist), I did not keep this journal for myself alone, but in hopes of making contact one day with a reader the way an astronomer cocks his great ear at the void, palpitating for the faint electronic evidence that we are not alone in the universe. What is this incessant scribbling if not a hankering for companionship, for that one dearest reader who will give me license without let or hindrance to, as Shakespeare says, "unpack my heart with words"?

This diary is a kind of self-portrait. It has little or nothing to do with the times in which it has been kept. For those concurrent events one would have to look elsewhere. My interest is in the language itself, for its own sake as well as for mine. Still, every word of it was written with one ear cocked toward the reader, to whose responses and feelings I am acutely sensitive. For me, too, the diary is a training ground for the exercise of wit. Only I cannot use it to purge myself of pain or resentment. That's the other side of recognition: shame. Your secrets are sure to be found out; your work will be used for other than your own intentions, a form of molestation. Yet one must live, and fame enables one to do so. In that sense it is an annuity.

The entries in my diary were written over a period of sixteen years, of which I present about half here, mainly from 1997 to 2001. During that time it has been my constant companion and comfort. I have kept it with diligence, the way one keeps a promise. When the day is dark, it is my fun to trouble the pages with a bit of foolery; when it is sunny, with an effort toward "nameless dread" like that expressed by Shakespeare's Queen in

Richard II: "Some unborn sorrow, ripe in fortune's womb / Is coming towards me, and my inward soul / With nothing trembles." Nor have these entries appeared on the page unanointed. I have edited them, selecting and rejecting words and paragraphs, rearranging the text in accordance with my writerly impulse. Editing them has been like buttoning a shirt, working each button into its hole, making sure you've got them straight. Each entry is a martyr that has been cut, seared, pitted, and flayed. Hardly a lazy, go-as-you-please enterprise. In the matter of strict chronology, I have preferred not to insist upon exact dates, but to give only years, if that, and sometimes even to reverse the calendar and let the past run up to me like an obedient dog.

A diary is perfect work for the elderly pen. There is a built-in coziness to the genre. The mind is curled up snugly on itself; no worry over such muscular matters as narrative drive, plot, irony, suspense—all those laborious considerations of a real writer. No need to invent words, insert them between quotation marks and follow with "he said" or "she said." A certain amoebic shapelessness prevails. No use in planning ahead, either, as the best entries are wrought *à la débandade,* after having left the ranks. Each entry in the notebook is a pseudopodium thrust outward to test the possibilities. Should the entry prove captivating, the whole organism is likely to pour itself in so that an essay or a story might happen. Only a small portion of such buds are developed; the rest are soon aborted.

But there is more to it than that. The very word *keep* evokes the idea of persistence, of not quitting. Other than the ledger of a business, a diary is the only book I know of that is kept. The word implies faithfulness to the task and preserving at least the appearance of privacy. The keep is the deepest part of the castle, where its treasures are held at time of siege. To keep a diary is to tend and marshal thoughts that might wander away the way sheep would were it not for the shepherd who keeps them. But my diary is hardly an intimate outpouring of the heart. Even when it affects informality it is self-protective and literary. The secrets are there, though, and best gotten at with a shovel. With all my pathetic attempts to be amusing, perhaps there will be one reader who will know that making fun is a way of hiding the sound of a small boy crying.

When I began this diary my idea was that it would be a way of "spying on myself from close up," in the words of Michel de Montaigne. I had meant for this diary to reveal the real Richard Selzer, a simple, ordinary man with the habit of writing down whatever he thought or did. Unlike my stories and essays, there would be no straining for effect. It would be free of the pomp of language and the vanity of the author. Simple, unadorned prose would be best. But almost immediately, I came face to face with the difficulty, if not the impossibility, of presenting myself to the public in a candid, orderly way without dressing up for the occasion. It was necessary that I make use of art and artifice, including metaphor, symbol, allusion, onomotopoiea, irony, and all the "airy medium of words" that make up the storyteller's instrument. In other words, I could not be other than what I am. My imagination is an especially demanding one; I have the duty and the desire to placate it.

Another difficulty was that of being absolutely factual, including only that which really happened. But I have always had no little trouble in differentiating fact from fiction in my life. Merely writing something down on paper makes it just as real to me as if it had taken place. In this I am supported by one of my literary-medical idols, Anton Chekhov, who advised the writer that if nothing exciting or interesting happened, he or she should make something up. The purpose was to amuse, entertain, and stimulate the reader. In other words, lying adds vitality to life. It is also fun. Many liars do it just for the pleasure it gives them. I confess that here and there I have "lapsed," but in every instance it was with the purpose of revealing a truth. The facts are only the facts; they lie on the surface of life. The truth goes deeper; it is "the real real that lies beneath the real."

1997

YALE'S STERLING MEMORIAL LIBRARY IS chock full of loonies, of whom I am one. Some are daily denizens, like me; others occasional drop-ins, depending on the weather. While one huddles in a corner with a shell-shocked faraway look, another reads the Turkish newspaper aloud. Still another, pricked by some devil, will leap from his seat in the Reading Room and shout an apostolic harangue until he is shushed, then rescued and defended by me. I am receptacular to these odd outscourings of the human race. They are argumentative, arrogant, often smelly and irritating, but it is the irritation of a grain of sand to an oyster: there is always the possibility of a pearl. Besides, they are my people, and how many of us would be thought sane were our lives to be examined closely? No, I despise them not, my fellow loonies, nor do they bore me, but are amusing and even interesting. As it is with physical deformity, so it is with my fellow loonies: their very irregularities become more remarkable than the principal fabric. This is not to say that they do not try one's patience. Today all seven of the loonies in my own personal "Ministry"—the ones in my care, so to speak—phoned in an upsurge of holiday mania. I spoke with each. "Not since Galahad . . . ," I told myself, when what d'you know, the phone rang seven more times—they each called again! At which I waxed wroth and meted out strokes of the birch. I have no heart, they said. And they are right, of course, though not for reasons within their ken.

It was from Father that I learned the beauty and power of the wound. It was from him that I discovered the beauty in what most people call ugliness or in fatigue. It is the tired voice that can be the most moving; it has endured; it has withdrawn from the ferocity of life. If all artists hear voices, why then the writing doctor is especially privileged: we hear the voices of our patients' bodies. For so long have I gazed at the human body with dilated pupils that now what gazes back at me is what by some might be called the soul. In such a vision the skin becomes the organ of recollection, remembering as it does the touch of a lover. A renal calculus is transformed into a bit of hard truth that lies hidden in the body. A perforated peptic ulcer is the hole through which pours all the rage and grief a man can harbor. And I have learned that the face is not the only doorway to the mind. I have seen sorrow more fully realized in a sacrum eaten away by decubitus ulcers, fear in the rapidly pulsating supraclavicular fossa of a neck, nakedness and shame in a kyphosoliotic spine, supplication in an arthritic wrist, and despair in the placement of a diabetic foot on the ground. Once I was informed by a man's kneecaps that he was ready to die; flashing blue lights, they teletyped the news that he was out of blood and oxygen. As soon as I received their cyanotic message, I summoned his family for a last visit.

In *Raising the Dead*, the account of my sojourn in the Valley of Death during a bout with Legionnaires' disease, I included the experience of my death and resurrection. Of course that didn't happen. I wrote it for the pleasure of writing it and for the effect it would have on the reader. In my defense, I did reveal later in the book that it was pure invention. The reviewers were not amused. "An act of pure mischief," it was termed. Had I been courageous I would not have confessed at all. I did so out of authorial cowardice. The real miracle was not my death and resurrection but the fact that the great majority of those who read *Raising the Dead* believed that it had happened. I admit that the mere writing of it has made it almost as real as anything that has happened to me. What I can say truthfully is that the patient released from the hospital after a close brush with death sees the world in a fresh way. It has been transformed by the possibility of having been lost. The ordinary becomes full of meaning. "A brighter emerald twinkles in the grass."

Here is what I wrote in my diary of 1993: "Thinking of *Raising the Dead*. How, at the beginning, it is true to life, but once under way the allegiance to art takes over. One crops here, shapes there, works in a metaphor; there will be elisions, asides, all the dishonesties of art. And worst, there will be an incident such as never took place—my death and resurrection—until the book has slipped its anchor to fact and is no longer the case history of a man with Legionnaires' disease. The solemnity and sadness of death have been transformed. Death itself will have been seized by the author and wrenched from the pages."

It is now more than five years later and I still reflect on it, but the horror has not chased me. I remember only the closeness of Death, that I was reconciled to it—welcomed it, even. That is the way with me: I have left behind all but one or two seemingly insignificant moments, but it is upon these that the whole of my life has been focused. I remain stupidly cheerful, by and large. Should an errant gust of melancholy stir the curtain, I think of that early morning when I was carried home from the hospital and put to bed in my own room. The cardinals, mockingbirds, and wrens were in full throat just outside the window. It was as if I were hearing their charivari for the first time. What a relief from the mortuary cooing of the pigeons that roost on the window ledges of the hospital.

It is five years ago that I completed the training and requirements for a shaman. This I did by falling ill, dying, and being resurrected (or so it has been alleged). A shaman is one who has been gravely ill and who is granted recovery if he promises cures to others. This he does not by mastering technique the way a medicine man or a doctor does but by taking upon himself the suffering of the patient and by intuition coming to understand it. The process is nothing more and nothing less than empathy.

Grandchildren—grand girls—Becky and Lucy slept overnight. I told ghost stories. They all but died of fright and joy. My wife, Janet, made me quit just short of irreversible mania. We baked a bread to calm ourselves down, then cut fat slices and slathered them with sweet butter and honey. The girls love me largely because I'm the only grownup who uses the word *poop* in a referential way, as in "Looks like dog poop to me." Today, though, Lucy, age five, said with immense hauteur: "Only babies say *poop*." I felt quite downcast all morning. Janet savored the moment rather too openly.

What with Sterling Library being closed for spring break—that crime against the institution of pedagogy—I have spent two days in the great hall of the Medical Historical Library. I sat there entirely alone in that vast paneled room lined with bookshelves, portraits, statues, and framed medieval manuscripts. The ceiling vaults perhaps forty feet up, arched with great, dark beams from which six large chandeliers are pendant. A railed gallery runs along three sides of the rectangle. Even higher is a clerestory of leaded glass. A huge fireplace is set in the far wall with on either side a padded banquette. Above the fireplace is a portrait of the sixteenth-century anatomist Andreas Vesalius, given by Harvey Cushing. Here one finds oneself in the continuum of medical history. The floor is of highly polished dark-stained wood, with a Persian carpet covering the area nearest the fireplace. The table lamps are old-fashioned: one must pull a chain; the lampshades allow the amber light to be reflected in the floor. I think of such lamps when I read, in Yoshida Kenko's *Essays in Idleness:* "The pleasantest of all diversions is to sit alone under a lamp, a book spread out before you, and to make friends with people of a distant past you have never known." On either end of the Persian carpet is a leather couch and its companion deep chair for snoozing. Here and there, punctuating the bookshelves, are statues of Vesalius, Ambroise Paré, Cushing, and the rest of the pantheon.

The books on the shelves are of the most tempting sort. I picked out one in Hebrew that offered the medical wisdom of the Talmud. Imagine my pride at being able to translate the title! Others are accounts of military campaigns by the surgeons who went along. It would be the death of me as a writer to return to such a paradise. And *tout seul*! Where in the world *is* everybody?

First day in East Rock Park. Saw, right away, a squadron of golden-crowned kinglets, all newly washed. As I walked on an isolated path, a shadow passed slowly over me. I looked up to see a turkey vulture *en glissade* only twenty feet over my head. Next, the rataplan of a large downy woodpecker, blazing red at the occiput. I followed the territorial call of the redwing blackbird and . . . there he was! In the river, a pair of mute swans, mallards. On the down side: altogether too many humans with their dogs.

Last year at this time, walking along a path in East Rock Park, I had one of my tilts: I saw myself coming toward me. Closer and closer the figure came until it seemed we two must collide or coalesce—whatever alter egos do when they come together. I felt an excitement as I hurried toward the lost Other, a sense that I would be made whole. At the last instant it was I who stepped aside while he strode manfully on without a hesitation in rhythm or a single backward glance. The same fragment left the park as had gone there.

Sitting in the library next to F.Q., not one of my Ministry of Loonies but a fanatical Christian evangelist. He is a graduate student whose subject is Milton. Suddenly N., a bona-fide loony (also a bona-fide genius of sorts), appeared at the table where I was working. As usual, he gave no sign of his presence—only "Dick!" barked out sharply so as to disturb everyone within earshot. It is the self-absorption of madness. They are incapable of any viewpoint save their own. I hustled him out-of-doors.

There were dark patches under his eyes, white inspissated saliva at the corners of his mouth, wrinkles, a wild look. He began by announcing that he had occult blood in his stool. I asked how he knew this. He just *knew*, that's all. I outlined a plan of investigation. That done, he rhapsodized over W. W. Jacob, an early-twentieth-century novelist and short-story writer. "He wrote an unadorned prose that you wouldn't like. Just told a great many cracking good stories." (Later I read one of these cracking good stories, "The Girl on the Barge." It is puerile, just right for someone stunted at the emotional age of twelve.) When he left I returned my attention to F.Q.

"One of your loonies?" he made bold to ask. I looked blank. "I thought so!" He has now identified three of the six, although I gave him no hint.

"The Redeemer liveth," I said, and held out my hands, palms up to show him the stigmata of the Crucifixion. Actually Dupuytren's Contractures—bunched scars that are the result of insidious fibrotic retraction of the palmar aponeurosis. *"Don't you know who I am?"* I added. F.Q. was not amused.

At age thirty-six he would have been handsome had not, in his youth, a satyr danced across his face leaving its hoofprints. Even now there are fresh pustules. Our gym lockers are next to each other so I know that the rest of his body is smooth and clean. Here is a man who must wear his corruption on the outside for all to see, while mine is kept hidden and all the more likely to be rotting away. F.Q. is a Christian in the narrowest sense. Devout, obsessed, humorless, he reads nothing that doesn't pertain. In addition to Milton, this includes Origen, Augustine, and the devotional poets John Donne and George Herbert. He is both anti-Semitic and homophobic. He is against abortion and in favor of capital punishment. He opposes the notion of female preachers. He is utterly lacking in caritas. Also, he is chock-full of lust, about which he can do nothing but writhe. He has behaved abominably toward a woman he caused to fall in love with him and then denied out of Christian morality. Sometimes we talk about sex.

"How," I asked, "can you continue to make love to your wife when you hate her so?"

"It's my duty. Says so in the Bible. It's better than abstinence, which leads to cancer of the prostate."

So, you might ask, why are we friends? I can only reply: *In my house there are many mansions.*

Report from the Ministry. With the resurfacing of G., the Ministry is again at full strength. G. used to phone up and speak to my answering machine for as long as two hours—fury, laughter, non sequiturs: brontoland. Once he phoned and spoke into the telephone for forty-five minutes while I was in the other room playing the piano. In between "Nina," "Vergin tutt' amor" and "Lascia me piange," I went back to the phone, said "Yes, yes" or "I see" or "too bad," then returned to the piano. He never noticed. He has been crazy behind my back for about a year. Presently he is full of rage, paranoid, with the entrenched delusion that any noise at all hurts his ears—hyperacousis, it's called: extreme sensitivity to sounds. His entire day is taken up with the avoidance of noise. It is not unlike F.'s "brain fatigue," which requires her to lie still all day in a dark room. With either, I avoid any suggestion or opinion. If G.'s ears are not hyperacute, his memory certainly is. He throws up to me remarks I made en passant fifteen years ago. One would think that somatic delusions would burn out in time, but no, these are necessary to G. and F., evidence that they are not mentally ill but are suffering from a "real" disease.

F. is perfectly content with her life, swallowing handfuls of vitamin pills and medication, resting her head, daydreaming. G., on the other hand, is furious, refuses any treatment, is wildly unhappy and lonely, and uses alcohol and marijuana in large quantities. V. also denies that he is ill, occupying himself with fantasies about women and writing "copy" for Ted Koppel's *Nightline*. He attends every free lecture offered at Yale but doesn't listen and more often than not walks out after a few minutes or, if he stays, peppers the speaker with outlandish questions. He loathes his family, who are alleged by him to have brought on his condition. In reality they are kind and deeply concerned for his welfare. V. eats nothing but Chinese vegetables and so is emaciated. For F., food is not part of the psychotic constellation. She eats everything. G. lives on bread and milk only.

Terrible as is their suffering (G. excepted), it is nothing compared to that of N. He is fully aware of his "madness"—an incapacitating Obsessive Compulsive Disorder that enforces solitude and misery. While the others are all of superior intellect, N. is just possibly a genius. In him there is a strong undercurrent of right-wing fanaticism and a fascination with guns.

It is fifteen years since I began this Ministry. What have I learned? That mental disease is the most refractory of all. Physical pain would be more bearable. The only thing I have to offer these people is my presence. I have befriended them, which is not the same as being their friend. They do not animate me, as friends do. Nor do they consider my needs. Periodically they fire me when I become the focus of their paranoia. Perhaps I have inadvertently said something dismissive? Not one of them is a jot better because of me. Not one is a jot worse, either. I cannot affect them in either way. I suppose that I do it out of some fascination with the abnormal, the pathological. I have a suspicion that Nature is more apt to reveal her secrets through her mistakes, those "incapable of perfectness" in the words of Francis Bacon.

And there is this from my diary of July 1993: "Ran into all six of my loonies on the street. Had to stop and chat six times. The flowerheads of the burdock will stick wherever they are thrown. You can pick them off your sleeve, but not your heart. And me in a hurry!

April and birdwatching time. I wear an old felt hat with a broad brim all around that has long since lost its stiffness and droops down on either side of my face like the ears of a basset hound. There are those in the park who train their field glasses on *me*. I can't blame them. Birds? What are *they*? Nary a one in East Rock. But who needs birds when one has a dozen floaters in his vitreous humor? No matter the vacancy of trees and sky, I walk the paths engulfed in movement and on the qui vive. I bring my own teeming migration.

Reading with great pleasure *Le collier des jours,* a memoir of childhood by Judith Gautier, daughter of Théophile. I am pleased that the French is quite manageable and I don't have to add up all the words that I don't know and take their average.

At Brown University I had just given my talk and was standing in the lobby among my tumultuous worshipers when across the open space I saw a woman standing at the head of the staircase, down which, sooner or later, I'd have to go, as the Men's Room was on the lower level. She appeared to be in her late thirties, with blond hair piled up and tied so that her long slender neck was naked. For a moment our glances met. Abruptly she turned away, but soon enough, as I knew it would, her gaze drifted back to where I stood among the students. Once again she looked into the beyond as though searching for someone. I knew better. Disengaging, I went as if to descend the stairs but instead stopped and gave her a smile of Annunciation. Moments later she had taken my hand and was smoothing it as though it were a piece of linen, examining the palm, running her finger over the hard-bunched scar of my Dupuytren's Contracture.

"What are you looking for?"

"Nothing. I wanted to hold the hand that performed those bloody deeds. And now writes with equal violence."

I opened my mouth to speak. What came out was a bright, melodramatic bray.

"I assure you, I'm harmless," I said.

"No. You are dangerous." When I laughed, she did too—but not really. Her eyes did not take part. I looked down at my hand still imprisoned in hers. "Take it away yourself," she said. "I won't give it back willingly."

When I climbed back up the stairs she was gone.

Several years ago, taking the train to Brown to give the Commencement Address, I eavesdropped on two young men, one of whom had been a "runner" for the Mafia and spent time in prison. He had grown up in Brooklyn and drifted into crime. "Let my mom down," as he put it. He was now a student at Brown. The other boy's family had befriended him, taken him into their home, and may have been responsible for his rehabilitation. The two mothers had spoken on the phone but had never met. The ex-con, a handsome light-skinned African American, recounted a scam he had pulled off not that long ago with the use of his credit card: he bought two thousand dollars' worth of clothes, brazened it out when questioned about it, and got away with it. A petty criminal without conscience or remorse. These two good-looking, smiling young men were on their way to Brown . . .

Easter Sunday. Janet and I walked to a Chinese restaurant for lunch: noodles, fish, eggplant, ice cream. Then I was off to the library, where I discovered it won't open until two, not even for me. So I sat on a bench in

Grove Street Cemetery and fell asleep in the sun. Awaking to find myself among the grateful dead, I took my pulse just to make sure.

I tried reading the letters of Evelyn Waugh and Nancy Mitford, two repellant characters devoid of both humanity and style. Such monsters! Also this month: *Sons and Lovers*, by D. H. Lawrence. This book, so loved by me at age sixteen, now makes me squirm. The nakedness of his characters, the obvious portrayal of himself in Paul Morel, the sexualized relationship between Paul and his mother, and all that reference to "the soul." I much prefer the body. Of course I have my limits. Montaigne describes the ballad of a cannibal who was the prisoner of another cannibal tribe. The soon-to-be-eaten-one tauntingly invites his captors to dine off him, for then they would be eating their own fathers and grandfathers. "This flesh," the man sings, "these muscles and these veins are yours, poor fools. Can you not see that the substance of your ancestors' limbs is in them? Taste them carefully and you will find therein the flavor of your own flesh."

Studied a hermit thrush with a rather sparsely speckled breast, brown back, pale abdomen, a reddish tail that bobs frequently, and no eye ring. Did the diary till 11, then perspired over a review I'm to write of Timothy Leary's *Design for Dying*, trying to find something good to say in the *New York Times Book Review* about this wretched piece of detritus. A young woman came up to me.

"Are you Richard Selzer?"

She told me that her class had read my essay "Skin," in *Mortal Lessons*.

"I loved it."

"I love *you*," I replied.

After lunch I went to see the cherry blossoms in Wooster Square, then to Long Wharf Theatre, where I met with Doug Hughes, who wanted to know whether I had any objections to a production of David

Rabe's play *A Question of Mercy,* based on my article, here. On the way back, I met one of my loonies, S.

"I am Saint Matthew," he said. "Josephus is my last name. I was also Sir Isaac Newton. He was born on Christmas day. Did you know that? All my hospitalizations are a Passion I suffer. About wings, they're not on the back for fun, they're at the bottom of your feet to propel you along. I will ascend soon, then you can have all my papers. I grant you full permission to give talks on my material."

Another triumph for modern psychiatry.

Morning coffee at Naples Pizza. Nearby, a young man with a shaven scalp, so naked as to present to view each ridge, plate, and suture of his skull, inion and all. I fought down the urge to go up and rub it for good luck. From the rear, with his features hidden, it gave the look of a death's head. Close peering revealed the ghost of a tonsure where the bitemporal and occipital follicles remained, the hair having been mowed to achieve uniformity. Among the balding it is no longer à la mode to scrape the remains of one's hair across the head so as to conceal as much skin as possible. Here, I thought, is a man wounded by baldness who has taken destiny by the lapels, seized the affliction, and made it his own the way a martyr seizes for himself the kingdom of Heaven, displaying a virile, brown-tinted scalp. As hair free as he was, his companion had little else *but,* with great jungles of it and isthmuses connecting an abundant cranial, mandibular, and supralabial acreage. I would not have been surprised had a Baltimore oriole poked its head out, taken a few turns about the man's head, and flown gratefully back into the nest.

Mornings of bliss, birding with my son Doon (Larry) in East Rock Park. We have chosen to avoid the conviviality and statistics of the Bird Club and have set out on our own. Can there be any pleasure greater than for a man to go birding with his son during the warbler migration? All the back trails up and down the mountain were ours and ours alone. With Doony's sharp eyes and split-second hand-eye coordination, I am *all' ombra del Signor*. He spots the bird, identifies it, and with all the patience of Aeneas carrying old Anchises points it out to me. Now, with rapidly failing vision and a late-born clumsiness, I see only half of what he shows me; the other half I pretend to see. The park itself is preternaturally gorgeous, with sheer cliffs, waterfalls, stone steps, a meandering river, footbridges, islands, gullies, hills both steep and sloping, overlooks with panoramic vistas, and more. On the ground, wild columbine, Dutchman's breeches, rare magnolias, even rarer yellow wild rose.

The Renaissance painter Luca Signorelli lost his beautiful, beloved son, who was killed in Cortona, the artist's hometown. With neither sigh nor tear but with intense concentration he copied the body of his dead son to keep him forever before his eyes, his creation for the second time. This is the basis for a story I plan to write in Italy, when I'm there giving my course on writing.

My dear Iraqi friend Saad visited at the library. Saad is a Muslim saint if ever there is one, with his sheikh's countenance and that whiff of the desert he emanates. His soul will simply not stay out of sight: every now and then it peeps out and is visible. His laughter is sudden and prolonged; when he weeps, it is for the world. He is utterly without egotism. He doesn't declaim, but murmurs in a soft voice that is more song than speech. He told me that at age thirteen he was betrothed to a seven-year-old girl with whom he shared his childhood. Then came degeneration of his hip, years in a Russian hospital, multiple surgical procedures, and a lifetime of pain. From Iraq he fled to France, where he met his American wife, who is a physician—she of whom he has never spoken to me. Today, for the first time, I told him of the esteem in which I hold him and the love that I have for him. I asked him never to change, but to always be Saad, at which he placed an arm around me as if to hug. I suspect that Saad knows personal unhappiness—I have never asked, he has never said, nor have we spoken of mine.

Awoke to the sound of warblers in the trees about the house. Raced through toast, coffee, and ablutions so as to get to the park early, only to find that my field glasses had disappeared from my car. Doubtless a thief in the night. Is there a deflation sorrier than that of the birdwatcher whose glasses are stolen at the height of the warbler migration? Just then my son Jon phoned, listened to my plaint, and said coolly, "You've still got your eyes." I disinherited him on the spot, then I kicked and swore my way to the library. Nor was my philanthropy returned to me by reading the last chapter of *Whitman and the Romance of Medicine*, Robert Leigh Davis's book on Whitman's hospital days, in which he couples Whitman and me under the rubric of homoerotic healers!

Walking on Hillhouse Avenue across from Saint Mary's Church, I hear a woman calling out from her car.

"Hey! Honey! Excuse me, Hon!"

I go to the window.

"You got a quarter for two dimes and a nickel? I need the meter."

We make the transaction. She is fat and blowzy and sits in a miasma of sweet perfume. A great deal of blond hair seems immovable.

"Gotta go to church. I'll pray for you, too, Honey. What's your name?"

"Dick."

"I'll pray for you, Dick."

I watch as she unpacks herself from the car, gives her skirt a purposeful twitch, and climbs the steps to Saint Mary's in the tiniest high-heeled gold slippers this side of Paradise.

≈

East Rock Park in the rain. Yellow-rumped warbler, Parula, waterthrush, redtail hawk, the wet lunacy shared by a straggle of cronies. I have just bought new field glasses to replace those stolen from my car. The new ones are Nikon 8 × 40 Naturalist 4 (whatever any of that means).

What with the blurring of my vision, to say nothing of the constant slow vermification of my muscae volitantes (floating concretions in the vitreous humor), the world has become out of focus in fact as well as in fancy. Everything is suffused with indistinction and peopled by phantoms. It is rather like swimming beneath the surface of a stagnant pond teeming with schistosomes, snails, *Dracunculus medinensis,* and whatever other parasites. Whereas before this gave me cause to shudder at the prospect of blindness and the "uncertainty" of the real world, I have lately embraced my affliction in hopes of spiritual reward. In the shifting haze, I find numerous pregnant possibilities. It is an adaptation that a writer can make and that a surgeon, say, cannot. In such a discarnate, "flow-y" state, bottles tilt and my toothbrush floats in the air, moving to and fro in a ghostly parody of its earthly raison d'être. In short, it is the ideal milieu for the artist. For instance: in such a "spiritual" state it is easier to commune with the dead. Only this morning I had a long chat with my paternal grandmother, Sophie—in Yiddish!—in which she admitted to me that my father, Julius, had not been sired by the same man as his two older siblings. I allowed as how I had figured this out while she was still alive.

≈

Let this date be known as the one on which I first saw the mourning warbler, a "life bird" for me and for that clutch of the blest who stood near the covered bridge in East Rock Park and gazed, at first in wild surmise, then in jubilation at the small bird with a pale-blue head and a black stripe on its breast, otherwise brown. Imagine the hosannahs and the instant camaraderie that bloomed in the Presence. "Cheery, cheery, cheery," sang the mourning warbler. "You bet!" we replied.

Met loony N. in the library. He was looking even more haunted, gaunt, and tormented than usual. He seems to be drowning in a sea of symptoms of a rare and relentless nature, each one a mystery. He says that he is exhausted from lack of sleep because of the colonic gas which builds up when he assumes a horizontal position. Many doctors have tried and none has succeeded in establishing an etiology. For his flatulence I prescribed a cat to place on his belly at night as a living compress. This was not well received. Now he has injured his foot by mere walking—a fascial inflammation, he says, controlled by proper and precise binding up by a podiatrist. He walks on tiptoe. Despite his abject despair, once engaged on Blake he discoursed with the same old brilliance while keeping, I noticed, his right eye closed at all times. He said that my observations on Blake's *Jerusalem* and the dance were new and worthy of pursuit. I asked him to attend the Blake exhibition at the Yale Art Gallery, then give me his impressions, but I think that not necessary. Already he knows more about Blake than anyone. It is stunning to watch that photographic memory click in. He agreed to see the paintings.

There is a profound difference between Blake and Michelangelo in that Michelangelo fondled even as he carved. The lust of the artist was the engine that drove his chisel. Not so with Blake, in whom whatever sensuality there is has been damped and replaced by the sanctification of the flesh. He has floated free of the carnal. Michelangelo's figures, though divinized, are nothing *but* erotic.

Dreaming of the lovely past week of birdwatching in East Rock with Doon. A blizzard of beaks and feathers blew into my eyes and ears all week long. Even my thoughts took wing. Eighteen varieties of warbler in as many minutes! And five of each! Doon quite marvelous—so patient with me, making sure that I saw every bird. Even when I couldn't find one, I lied and said that I had, to give him the filial pleasure. To have such a son! Sometimes I trained the field glasses on *him* instead of a bird and let my heart swell.

As for the trip to Tuscany, it *looms*. It's like a locomotive with poor Selzer tied to the railroad tracks. Yes, I know . . . it's a far cry from Chekhov's journey to Sakhalin, but still . . . I can only hope that on the appointed day (May 30) "they" will have paved the sky smooth and ironed all the ruts from the clouds, and I shall pray to Aeolus that he might blow from the west. Once having arrived at the Rome airport I'm to betake myself to the railroad station, board a train, change to another, and leap off as it slows down but doesn't quite stop at the village of Bonconvento. There, *pace, pace, mio Dio,* I am to be picked up and brought to the farm. My blood congeals at the prospect. To add to the usual level of self-loathing, I've not yet dug the garden to make it ready for dill, basil, and lettuce. Nor will I.

I'm just back from a trip to Springfield, Illinois, where I gave a Commencement speech, or rather seized and rassled the lectern to the stage floor. I was unaccountably teary and had to gulp a lot during the talk, can't say why. The sentimentality of old age? Masked depression? The sleepless night? I asked to be taken to Lincoln's tomb. It was grand, even imperial I should say, with a tall obelisk of white granite and numerous bronze statues. On top there is an open "deck" where you can read the names of all the states carved into the base of the obelisk. With the gravest

ill-taste, the names of the states were abbreviated. For example, ARIZ. Or
N. MEX. Those carved periods are surely offensive. Only Ohio, Utah, and
Iowa escaped this indignity. Such is the tomb of our greatest president and
most eloquent statesman. When I remarked upon this to my hosts, no one
had noticed. Take care, America, lest you end up a vast plain of salt.

My short story "Whither Thou Goest" was the talk of the place. Also
my poor little "Raccoon," of all things. The trip was worthwhile if only to
restore my flagging self-confidence at the podium. All the audiences were
most responsive—I needn't have fretted. Also, the pleasure of meeting my
host, Patrick Persaud, a Guyanese of Indian heritage, a Heidegger student, phenomenologist, and New Testament scholar who reads biblical
Greek. I peppered him with questions. What did Jesus mean when he said
to Mary Magdalene, "Touch me not, for I have not yet risen"? Why did
he tell his mother at Cana, "Woman, what have I to do with thee?"
Patrick has such a sensible approach to the Scriptures and was hugely
patient with me.

There is, of course, a deep connection between "Whither Thou Goest"
and the book of Ruth, which is part of what we talked about. There was a
famine in the land of Judah, and so Elimelech (God is King), a man living in
Bethlehem (House of Bread), brought his wife, Naomi, and two sons to the
land of Moab. Elimelech died, and the two sons married Moabite women,
one of whom was Ruth. When the two sons also died, leaving Ruth alone
with Naomi in Moab, Naomi learned that the famine in Judah had passed and
she decided to return there. She urged Ruth to remain in Moab, but Ruth
refused to part from her mother-in-law. "Whither thou goest," she said, "I
will go. Thy land shall be my land. Thy God, my God." When they arrived
in Judah, in dire poverty, the barley harvest was in progress, so Naomi
advised Ruth to go gleaning in the fields of a man named Boaz to avoid
starvation. Boaz, a wealthy kinsman of Elimelech, saw Ruth, was attracted to
her, and took her for his wife, also marrying out of his faith. From this
marriage the descent was to Jesse, who was the father of David. Ruth was
thus the great-grandmother of David.

In my "Whither Thou Goest," in which a woman decides to listen to the heart of her deceased husband as it beats in the chest of another man, I was struck by the connection between gleaning in the fields and the soft words of husbandry and the soil—*harvest* and *transplantation*—that are used to describe the surgical procedures in relocating the organs of one person into the body of another, as was done to the young husband of my heroine. The idea for the story came to me from a small article in the *New York Times* that told of the murder of a man and the ensuing placement of seven of his organs into seven recipients. At first I was undecided about how to tell the story. I might have told it from the perspective of the physician who asked permission of the wife to retrieve the organs of her brain-dead husband. I might have told it from the point of view of the heart itself. In the end, I chose to tell it from the wife's point of view. The state of widowhood baffles her and keeps her from going on with her life until she locates the heart and hears it beating again. When the story first appeared in a magazine, the editor changed the title from "Whither Thou Goest" to "Follow Your Heart." Of course this was done without my permission. The beautiful biblical allusion was destroyed.

Yesterday's lunch at Mory's turns out to have been an examination for the Boys Friendly. This morning Maynard Mack phoned with the invitation to join their Monday lunch club, consisting of Maynard, Louis Martz, Eugene Waith, Claude Rawson, Murray Biggs, George Hunter, and Fred Robinson. I was, he said, overwhelmingly approved. So I shall join Mory's in order to do so. The Boys Friendly has been in existence for more than fifty years. Since the "table down at Mory's" holds only eight people, one member has to die before another is taken in. I am the replacement for Professor John Pope, a scholar of Old English who died at the age of ninety-five not long ago. Just so is one eased into the Establishment willy-nilly. Still, I'm honored to be confrères with such eminence. Of the seven, five are well into their eighties, so I shall relish the rarity of youth, no matter how relative.

In Italy for my week-long course on writing. One day the class and I went to Siena. While they wrote, I visited the duomo, a black-and-white-marble cathedral second only to the duomo at Milan in the matter of ugliness. All those alternating stripes of black and white marble laid transversely—the genius spent on it makes the monstrosity all the more scandalous, what with the zebraic God that dwells therein. I cannot partake in its achievement, the false dignity of its very great age notwithstanding (it is thirteenth-century Moorish). Just outside and down the hill, the Campo is infested with tourists. Tiny weeds and wildflowers are upthrust between the pink bricks, their fate to be trampled by alien feet. Close it for three months and you'd have a lovely meadow. As for ornate white marble fountains, give me the wooden pump handle of a backyard well.

So now you know into what a green grump I have fallen. I rather enjoy it. I'd no idea how much fun it is to put everything down!

Step inside the vast dark nave of a cathedral or duomo. It hints of the black vastness of the universe itself. A pagan moss grows over the damp walls. From high above comes the cooing of pigeons. Now and then one swoops low. Only the gilded statuary, the brass fittings are bright and gleaming. Come closer to transept, apse, altar and see that Mary is deep in grief, that Jesus is suffering great pain, and that Joseph is exhausted. You are called to this church to sympathize with the Holy Family—to feel, if you can, their suffering. You are also asked to admire the art and craft with which they have been rendered for your veneration. The air is filled with incense, there is the flickering of votive candles, the echo of footsteps on a stone floor, the unearthly sound of Gregorian chant and the clicking of beads. It takes a stern grasp on the natural to resist such persuasion, but as for ever converting to Catholicism, it would be with all the enthusiasm of a small boy inching himself into the cold end of a swimming pool. I am put off by the blatant theatricality of the whole display, to say nothing of the multitude of infantilized saints, each of whom has upended nature with miracles, then died young and horribly.

About Tuscany, there is only one word: beautiful, something to behold at every turn. But I'm relieved to be home. The travel is grueling, for me, at least. While I wrote not a word, I did make friends with some women: two in their twenties, one a Botticellian Venus who, in a gesture of exquisite generosity, offered to make love to me! How wise (and how stupid) of me to decline, à la Chekhov. I also drew close to Joel Meyero-witz, who is probably the most sensitive, holiest man I know—a great artist. I loved just being near him, listening to him talk about cameras, lighting, and street photography. The workshop itself? No writers, but two or three will surely publish, so what do I know?

In the Monastery of Monte Oliveto, about half an hour from the farm where I stayed in Tuscany, I saw a cloister plastered with the frescoes of Luca Signorelli. It was a coincidence that I embraced. I always do wher-ever they come up. And so I am well into a short story about that painter. So far it is still embedded in the journal notebook. But I am enjoying the process after a lapse of what seems like years.

I am in at the library writing letters, hoping to begin some real writ-ing again. The Signorelli frescoes were a disappointment, so perhaps I shan't do the story I had planned around them. We'll see what comes to mind.

The Men's Room at Sterling Library is a charmless subterranean stone box with on one side a row of stalls and on the other six sinks and six urinals. Above the bank of urinals is a recessed window that on rare occasions admits a pale ray of sunlight. It is of troubled glass not meant to be looked through. The outside of the window is protected by a wire mesh into which ivy has grown. Standing at a urinal, you can look up to see the waggling of its paltry leafage. Now this is what I call true vegetable courage. With five million books upstairs, it is in the Men's Room of Sterling Memorial Library where Beauty and Truth are to be found.

❧

Arrived at Chautauqua in a state of utter defeat. I am here to lead a week-long writing workshop. A ghastly journey. Three-hour wait in Washington, failure to be met in Buffalo. Waited there for an hour, as I didn't know the name of the limousine company. Many useless phone calls to closed offices and answering machines. Just about to go back home when there he was. The driver rose above my scalding assessment of his character, lineage, and ineptitude. Four stops to take on other Chautauquans with whom I declined to exchange a single word, lest it be one I'd have to eat tomorrow. I arrived at Fernwood (so-named for the many hanging baskets of that vegetable on the porch), the cottage whose third floor was to be mine for the week, to find a bottle of Absolut in the kitchen, courtesy of my hosts. I could have wept. Actually did, I think. After three ounces on the rocks, a hot bath and a bowl of soup, I felt all better.

Sunday, endless Sunday. From every porch, the melancholy sound of hymns, earnest, off-key, fuzzy at the edges where the congregants don't keep together. "Blessed Be the Ties That Bind" and "Fairest Lord Jesus" waft through the ancient maples like the bombination of bees in a lime tree. Then, at the end: "Hallelujah" and "Hosannah—He Comes!" With that, the music is no longer fuzzy, it is clarified.

There is a great preponderance of elderly here at Chautauqua. Many must be hand-led or wheeled. Creaky, given to polite mumbling, so frank in their religiosity. Virtuous folks on the many paths—Lutheran, Congregational, Methodist—that converge on Heaven. And they are fat. Such hams and bellies and hocks to present on Resurrection Day, when "this very flesh (*ipso corpore*) will rise"—it could be a problem, an overloading of the system. Well, hush—needn't be so cynical. Their souls are visible. Mine is heavy-lidded and sleeping in, chock-full of vice. I must comfort myself with pen and notebook, like the littlest god. But there is the feeling of being herded here, there, everywhere, with hundreds waiting in line for free tickets to chamber music, the concert at four in the afternoon, the line formed at seven in the morning. And there is a self-congratulatory air about the place: one belongs to the best, one has figured out how to obtain and savor the finest poetry, music, drama, current events, lectures. In fact, the ballet aside, I've seen nothing first-rate.

A new pain, high under the left ribs, a sense of "crowding." Affected by stretching, position. Sat in a tub with some relief, only to have it recur. At least the first workshop is over. It was minimally enjoyable. I made a solemn oath never to do it again. Then the new pain returned. I have a fear of being sick here and a burden to my hosts. My hands do this, my feet do that without my telling them. I phoned Janet, just come home from strewing her friend Chris's ashes in New Hampshire. My being away gives her grieving space without restraint. I also phoned P.L., who has recovered from the surgery. Is he reading easier now? "Yes." So much in one word! My talk went well. I was paid all of fifty dollars. I have run out of vodka, so I must borrow a car and get to a package store.

The workshop is a roaring success, with everyone turning out good work. This is a full-time job: preparing and holding the daily class, conducting individual meetings, reading the work, and commenting. Not for me a vocation, but I enjoy the comradeship of the students, their obvious affection and appreciation. I have stopped attending any of the entertainments. The Program Committee takes dead aim at mediocrity and never misses, ballet and Brahms excepted. And me.

Agreed to be interviewed by V., one of my loonies, his speech slurry from medication, all but unintelligible. Unkempt, needing a shave, yawning, corpulent but peaceful, the grimaces of tardive dyskinesia notwithstanding. We sat on the back porch of the Lizzie (the Elizabethan Club at Yale) while he posed mystifying issues. "Can pain protect other people?" "Are there good qualities that cause pain?" I'm quite sure he knew what he meant. Though I meandered around the topic, he wrote down every word I said on a yellow legal pad. The reason for this interview is also mysterious. I but acquiesced.

Struggling to write the Tuscan story, I feel that I'm on the verge of solving it. Twenty-five years ago I'd have just sat down and written it. I made the mistake of groaning within earshot of Janet. "You don't have to write it, you know." As if it were a dish of oatmeal that I didn't have to eat!

I recall a dinner party several years ago in honor of Mr. Justice Blackmun. My tablemate, a professor of law at Yale, assured me that he never once kept a secret from his wife. Did that apply to the private remarks of his clients? Absolutely! He would not accept a client who did not understand beforehand that his case would be shared with the lawyer's wife. Not only is this the height of stupidity, it is reckless to aerate a marriage with perfect candor. The weather soon turns inclement.

The Tuscan tale is finished. I have now only to name it. Report on matters of *fundament*al importance: still sore and inflamed; can't sit. Maimonides wrote standing up—I may just have to follow his example.

Ice storm such as to confine me to the house, but not before a convincing fall down the front steps and a sore wrist. Whenever I cannot go to the library I become quite evangelical—without knowing where to lay my head. It gives but the faintest inkling of homelessness.

As for my lineage, once having landed on the continent of North America, both my grandparents—my father's mother and my mother's father—never looked back. Not for them the nostalgia or rancor of the exile. They were late settlers, looking only toward a new life. They strove to shed the vestiges of the shtetl—the accent, the costume, even the ritual, until only humor, cynicism, and a taste for anarchy were left—but not pessimism, never that. And the cuisine. They simply could not forgo their latkes, chalupchas, varonigas, and gefilte fish. Man's heritage is most deeply rooted in the stomach. But whatever else may be cast off, memory cannot. It is unshuckable. Often enough I listened to it venting in the form of sighs. Food aside, the children were goyim, albeit goyim who could speak Yiddish when necessary. Whenever I would ask about life "over there," I was dismissed with a sniff of distaste or a shrug. "Never mind all that." So I don't know the name of the country from which they came, nor even the village. At least I know that Father was born in a village outside Odessa and that his mother grew cucumbers and sold them at an open market. Or did I make that up?

Awoke convinced that I am used up, not a dewdrop of imagination left, not a speck of fairy dust. It's gone, and I shall be a lump. Time was (yesterday) when all I needed was a pen and notebook. But that was long ago (yesterday). What is there left? Just the old hankering after what never comes. There is something ineffably pitiful about a seventy-six-year-old adolescent, still thumbing his nose at the "adult" world, still bent on shocking the bourgeoisie, reveling in the adoration of the like-minded and relishing the attention of the Establishment.

Presented "Pietà" to a packed house at the Medical School, a talk that I wrote originally for the Yale Art Gallery, where the beautiful Bavarian Pietà, sculpted out of wood, is on display. This anonymous work is the ultimate flower of the linden tree from which it was carved. It is the root as well, with the rich damp earth from which it was harvested clinging to the rhizomes. Whenever I go to the gallery I can almost smell it, which cannot be said for ivory or metal or any other material from which sculpture is made. In fact, here is a heresy if ever there was one: unlike this Pietà, Michelangelo's is a perfect, cold beauty. I do not feel the grief of the Mother. The passion is his, Michelangelo's. Perhaps it's the gleaming marble, a medium that hasn't the warmth or the evidence of having once been alive that are the attributes of wood. By the time this wooden Pietà was half carved, the sculptor could touch sorrow with one finger. That an emotion or idea can become visible and palpable—in ivory, clay, stone, *or* wood—is a matter of wonder to me. Had this Pietà been left among its worshipers, I doubt that anything of it would remain. Who could resist touching it? And with each touch a speck of the statue would depart on the fingers of the faithful. Over the centuries wells and declivities would have diminished the shape and size of the figures until they had been transmuted into pure reverence itself.

Time was when statues of the Pietà had an earthly purpose. They instructed illiterate worshipers about their faith. They told the beloved story to those who came to church and could not read. The statues were there to be venerated, adored, and, especially, prayed to. Not any more. Now they are looked at in curiosity and admiration as specimens of form that signify only themselves. The devotion that created them and the honor that was paid to them have long since fallen into disuse. Faith has been transmuted into Art. It is a comedown.

On second thought, it is not the statue itself that is venerable, it is the invisible that exists within it. This is true of all art, whether sacred or profane. There is the ineffable, of which you cannot speak or write. There is no language for it.

Is it possible that Providence, out of some hidden purpose, grants to certain people at charged moments a glimpse of what lies outside the precincts of the natural world? I think so. Such phenomena appear suddenly and vanish just as quickly, going out like a snuffed candle. Their appearance is neither for good nor for evil, but only to show themselves. I should think these "manifestations" or crossings-over occurred more often in ancient times, before civilization had dulled our receptacularity. In at least two stories I have tried to suggest another reality, an *otherwise* that lies beyond the boundaries of consciousness. Call it what you will— imagination, spirit, the god element—it is a not-to-be-rendered-precisely presence, always there but seldom perceived or recognized. One way to approach the mystery is through language. Another is via dream, meditation, trance. For some it is music that triggers the vision. For others it is prayer. In "Fetishes" and "Tillim" I have done it by use of epiphany—a sudden flash of revelation. It shares with the phenomenon of orgasm an erasure of the conscious mind in a flood of intense sensation, a something-not-ourselves but yet a something-lodged-within-us. It is both the quintessence of otherness and the quintessence of ourselves. The impossibility of defining this is apparent in the awkwardness of my language. I am quite sure *this* will not clarify anything. Perhaps there are things that human beings ought *not* to see?

In Aspen I appeared at an ethics conference that was solemn with argument and rejoinder. What ethicists have to learn is the difference between mystery and dilemma. A mystery may well be eternal and if so has every right to keep its secret. A dilemma is earthbound, mortal: one has an obligation to try to resolve it. Attendance at the conference included philosophers and theologians as well as doctors. For philosophy, I have the wrong-shaped head; for theology, I have too scrawny a butt: a big clerical ass and a German accent are essential. Besides, I may be the most unethical man in North America.

Returned last night from a week in Colorado still unable to use the computer. The print is too small, I don't do capital letters right, and that is going to be that until the Day of Resurrection. I gave nine presentations, for my sins, the last in a place called Beaver Creek, which, like Aspen, is characterized by beautiful geography and disgusting wealth. I met many fine people and was lionized unto coma. *What One Man Said to Another* was all over Colorado—I even signed a copy of it.

As for Cormac McCarthy's *Child of God,* I continue to be astonished by his mastery of language, his flamboyant style, his unerring and novel imagery. And I continue to be nonplussed by his egregious love of depravity and violence for its own sake. What a waste! All that great gift laid at the feet of cruelty. The necrophiliac scenes—just the idea of there being more than one!—are so disturbing as to be unforgettable. That scene wherein he leads the men into the cave and entraps them is marvelously wrought, as is the scene in the shooting gallery. McCarthy could have been the finest writer of our time, no question, but after all, this is literary jerking off. Sorry, I can't genuflect before this guy.

The trouble with modern literature is that there is too much of it, that *much* having to do with the word processor. Facilitation is almost always detrimental. Art ought to be laborious. In a better world a writer would be permitted to publish only those works written with a pen of his own making, the way that an oboist must cut his own reed or else remain unheard. It is no great feat to make a pen; a walk on the beach at molting time with a penknife to sharpen the quill is all. Considering the mechanical ineptitude of most writers, even so small a task would serve to suppress the peristalsis of publishing.

I can't help but be struck by the banality, the ordinariness of my life. It's what I both despise and count on. Small, silly misunderstandings are what propel me from one day to the next, most often fueled by the adage *Least said, soonest mended.* It's the slogan of the timid. I am the cracked plate that stays intact by some fragile cohesion that ought not to be examined too closely. What has given me the greatest pleasure is not love but writing: gathering up the words I find lying all over like leaves, seedlings, feathers, pebbles. I brush them off, set them down in a line just so, and wait for them to sing. Sometimes after writing a sentence I sit back, lick the cream from my snout and purr. End of myself.

There is more than one advantage to having been a surgeon before becoming a writer. It is in the matter of discipline. If it can be said of any medical specialist that he is disciplined, it can be said of a surgeon, who must screw his courage to the sticking point at any hour of the day, no matter the other demands on his life. The surgeon-turned-writer can transfer this discipline into the act of writing. He doesn't need to put it off until the last moment. No need to get up and sharpen a pencil, take a drink of water, make a phone call, all of which "nesting" is like the dog who turns round and round before lying down on the rug with a huff and a thump. The surgeon is always ready.

I had a friend who was the world's leading authority on Mayan civilization. One of my former students, now an editor at a publishing house, contracted with the professor to write a book on the subject. An advance was paid, then a year and a half went by during which no word had passed between editor and author. When the editor finally phoned to ask how the project was going, he was greeted with a burst of outrage that the editor had dared to intrude upon him, and a warning not to do it ever again. A number of years went by, again with no communication between them. When the editor learned that a conference on Mayan culture was being held in Boston, he decided to attend, and there he found the professor surrounded by a circle of admirers to whom he was handing down wisdom. The editor then decided to risk another episode, only this one in public.

"Ah, Professor," he said. "And how is the book progressing?"

"Famously, famously," replied the old professor. "Nothing down *on paper* yet, mind you." And that was to be that.

Unbeliever that I am, I am ever on the trail of the marvelous. But sometimes it's hard to keep a straight face in the presence of Great Religious
Art. In *The Death of Saint Francis* by Giotto at the Yale Art Gallery, the
newly dead and laid-out saint is surrounded by monks, priests, and crip-
ples. Four friars, one at each hand and foot, are seen kissing (or licking?)
the wounds of the stigmatic. A knight, Saint Jerome of Assisi, is shown
lifting aside the saint's shirt and inserting two fingers into the spear
wound in his side, inserting them right up to the proximal interphalangeal
joints! He looks for all the world like an old-time surgeon probing for a
bullet, or a gynecologist doing a pelvic examination. Is he reenacting
Christ's invitation to Thomas to rid himself of doubt, or does he act out of
some dark, private preoccupation?

Letter to Peter Josyph. Dear Matisse—I address you so because I am
certain that by now you and he are one and the same person. That is what
happens when you write someone down on paper. There is a gradual
transmigration until writer and character meld, fuse, merge, and are one.
This has happened to me any number of times. I am presently writing a
"character sketch" of a man I never liked, and what d'you know?—it's
me! I surely do wish one of those publishers would see the light and bring
out novel no. 1. You know what a debased *industry* that is. One can do
nothing about it. Only rejoice that they don't throw us in jail for writing.
Doubtless that too will transpire.

D'accord, I've been enjoying my sabbatical from the podium. You can't
imagine what bliss it is to have no deadline and no destination. Only the
library, the Lizzie, the gym, and home. That's my *piccolo mondo*, and I
love it. I'm presently writing that character sketch and thinking about

Saint Peter and Thomas Eakins's *The Veteran* for a gallery talk I'm giving in May. I may write it as a dialogue between the two.

I am not going to renew my subscription to Long Wharf Theatre. The season so far, with one exception, has been awful. And David Rabe's adaptation of my *A Question of Mercy* is still to come. I may put an announcement in the *New Haven Register:* "Dr. Richard Selzer apologizes to the citizens of New Haven for the forthcoming annoyance of *A Question of Mercy.*" I surely do hope everyone comes to their senses about this play. I can't fathom it, really. I may have to take the veil and get me to a monastery for the spring season.

If it is true, as Oscar Wilde said, that sensual pleasures wreck the soul, mine should be shipshape and spanking. Never mind. I have waxed rich. My flocks and my herds have been increased by the addition of a chest of viruses. The way they tunnel among my lungs! Each time I cough, the scampering, the squeaks! Until all is quiet again . . . hideously quiet.

Phone call from one Peter Hinkle, whose "crushed" hand he says that I repaired back in 1964—bones, tendons, pins, skin graft, and all. He had been Yale's champion javelin thrower and broke all the records, he told me. He calls now, thirty-four years later, to express his "eternal gratitude." He is throwing again and "quite well." For all of which I haven't a shred of recollection. I told Janet he had said that I was the only surgeon in America who could have saved his hand, then I waited for her comment. It came: "He's obviously not heard of Bob Chase." Bob is my beloved chief resident and a truly great hand surgeon, of whom I refuse to be jealous.

Janet left for France. I prepared the going-away dinner: borscht, frican-deau, roast potatoes, horseradish. I said, "Imagine sitting down at the table and being served horseradish made with your husband's very own tears." We exchanged fugitive smiles until it was time to go to the airport. Once back home, I lowered every blind and windowshade but one, turned off all the lights, let voice mail take care of the phone, and sat in the one un-shielded window to converse with the moon. All this to discourage the pilgrimage of women who cannot believe how extremely married I am, and of the men who pant to speak with me, to become writers, or to speak with me *about becoming writers*. Having transformed Saint Ronan Terrace into a hermitage with only its one old gnome left, I lay down in bed, pulled the whole terrace over me like a blanket, and went to sleep.

1998

IT IS TWELVE YEARS SINCE I retired from surgery. There are times even now when the nostalgia for the operating theater becomes painful. Then I am drawn to the Yale Medical Library, where in the beautiful Cushing Rotunda there is a perpetual display of antique surgical instruments all bristling with potential. Here are stone-scoops, trochars, rasps, lancets, fleams, reamers, and scrapers, each meant to incise, dissect, extract, disimpact, detorse, and otherwise disturb the status quo of the body. The palms of the old sawbones itch; he all but neighs and stamps like a retired warhorse at the smell of battle and blood. But I am a child of my times, and those times are past. Nowadays one manipulates chopsticks through a tiny aperture and calls it surgery. Or inserts a fiberglass wire into a blood vessel until it reaches the heart, or thrusts one down the throat all the way to the ampulla or vater and beyond. Where is the passion, the heroism, the drama in that?

In 1679 a famous headsman in Prague watched a team of surgeons replace a head he had just severed from the shoulders of a young criminal. The lad was kept alive for half an hour, it is written. Panurge did better than that with his transplant. The recipient torso went on to live out his normal lifespan, or so Dr. Rabelais hath related. Why make so much of the head? It is there, said Galen, for the express purpose of holding up the eyes so that they might see farther in pursuit of food and mate: the head as lighthouse of the body.

As in the surgeon, so in the headsman, it was dexterity that counted. Sureness of stroke was all. And doubtless, as a profession, headsmen were no less arrogant and self-flattering than we are. Perhaps it would be pro bono publico to invite the public to attend surgical operations, as was the custom at beheadings. Then any bungling or botching would be met with the derision it deserves. I imagine a TV show in which two surgeons are pitted against each other, their identical operations being performed then and there. At the end, the studio audience will vote yea or nay, and the loser will be expected to turn his scalpel upon himself.

❧

Arrived home from Salt Lake City, where I had given a talk to a long line of the mentally moribund, with my own nerves in tatters after a horrible journey. "I missed you so much!" is the general expression, for I had been *hors de consultation* for all of three days. The outcry is surely meant, but it is also a veiled accusation of abandonment. Where to begin? N. is suing two doctors over two separate experiences. During a herniorrhaphy, the ilioinguinal nerve was caught in a suture, giving him continuous testicular pain—of this he is certain. Then there is the gastroenterologist who must have perforated his bowel two years ago, as he has had excessive flatulence ever since. He is sure there's an occult abscess. Do I remonstrate? Then I am part of the "medical conspiracy." Do I say nothing? Why, then, am I not equally outraged? He is thin, pale, haunted, with wisps of gray at the temples and a rare fugitive smile that, finding its perch upon his features uncomfortable, soon flutters off.

Next in line is B.T., a graduate student who has his own problems. "Yale is crushing my spirit. I'm unbearably lonely." What's wrong, he wonders. "I'm young, handsome, fun to be with." All of which is true. Why then can't he find someone to love? Because five minutes in his company reveals the despair and depression that would engulf and smother a companion. He has been diagnosed as manic-depressive, takes a quantity of medications, claims to have an addictive personality. Still, he has given up smoking, does daily exercise, and drinks no more. That he is gay doesn't make his plight any easier, despite what the sociologists say. He hunts me down at the library each day. I hesitate to let him come too close for fear of doing him harm.

And then there is P.P., a computer repairman I met in the stacks. He defines the term *nebbish* as used by our forefathers: small, pink, rabbity, paranoid, and hypochondriac. At age forty he lives with his parents and a single sister. His pleasure is the theater, which he attends in New York. And these, N. excepted, aren't even my *real* loonies. Nor can I take them on. In my house there are just not *enough* mansions. The incidence and intensity of public madness has risen, it would seem. I, too, am madder than before.

Went to the Educated Burgher for coffee and a muffin, was followed in by V., one of my loonies.

"Buy me an orange?"

"My pleasure."

V. seems calm, regimented, *medicated*. He'd attended a lecture about my work and told me that he stayed until the end. I congratulated him. He accused me of ingratitude for not attending myself, and smiled to himself at having captured me at last. When I rose to leave he reached for my sleeve. "I haven't seen you for so long." Medication can only do so much.

Already, at ten o'clock in the morning, the fatigue gathers as if it were the dark middle of the night. Oh for an amulet to ward it off!

It is a paradox that I am both a religious writer and a skeptic. Chatting with a birdwatching crony about religion, I told him that I had been given the grace of unbelief. All that is left to me of Judaism is a palate for what my brother Billy used to call Jewfood and a sprinkle of Yiddishisms. Other than that I'm washed as clean of it as the Holy Ghost, and would be up for grabs by the Catholics were it not for the saints, angels, pope, and celibacy of the clergy, none of which I can stomach. Add to that the general hypocrisy about sex and Confession and you have the reason I am beyond the pale of that otherwise quite satisfying faith, replete with bells, incense, and statuary—and the certainty that God is always right there for you when you need him. Oh yes, there is the unedifying penchant of cardinals to bless their favorite baseball teams at the opening game! That is why, I told my friend, I sin without guilt, tell no beads, and venerate no idols. No, I do not pray in any conventional sense, as I do not believe there is a God to receive prayer. But I do pray (if that's what you call it) *out of earshot,* and ask my heart, "Why did I laugh tonight?" (Keats), and other difficult questions. And I am attentive to everyone and every living creature, just as a nun includes all humankind in her prayers. That means listening and beholding with all of my might.

In Surinam there lives a four-eyed fish called, with utter disregard for the mellifluous, *Anableps tetrophthalmus.* In the muddy waters of the creeks, an armada of these small submarines will swarm over the tidal flats. The water is cleft by triangular wakes. At the forward apex of each wake a pair of tiny periscopes glides. They are unique among animals in that their eyes are divided horizontally into two halves. The upper half is so refracted as to see clearly in the air. The lower half is focused for seeing in water. As it glides along in search of food, or to watch out for danger, *Anableps tetrophthalmus* sticks the upper half of its eyes out into the air while, with the lower half, it performs these functions below the surface of the water. I know of another creature with similar faculties: the artist.

I am having all sorts of "loony" problems. M. is a forty-seven-year-old Chinese-Canadian psychotic who had been my student in a writing seminar one summer at Yale. As her behavior was too bizarre for inclusion in the class, I suggested that she remain silent and she and I could meet privately. This was interpreted as a keen romantic interest on my part. Since then she has written me countless letters, sent tapes, been hospitalized for three months, and lost her job as teacher of English to Chinese immigrants. She's coming from Canada for a day. Imagine! She'll take the night bus to New York City, stay there overnight, train to New Haven, and check in at the Holiday Inn. Next morning I pick her up, listen to the manic babble till after dinner, then bye-bye. I feel lucky to be getting away with only one day of it. But I did lay down the law. The poor creature is awfully sick and has been for twenty years.

I took my grandchildren Emmy and Danny out in back of the house. The Bamboo Forest planted twenty years ago by their father has flourished in fact and myth. Some of the canes are forty feet in height. At night they creak like the shrouds of a sailing vessel with new canes sprouting underfoot. The little grove has taken on a magical property. The witch who lives in the Taft Mansion does not dare to trespass here, so no need to worry. (Just today I peered through my field glasses and saw her in a window.) The path that runs through the Bamboo Forest leads directly to the Magic Tree, a gigantic tripartite weeping beech that has been the source of much wildness of imagination *chez nous*. The tree is composed of metamorphosed elephant, giraffe, and alligator. We have each ridden on the elephant's trunk, mounted the back of the alligator, and petted the giraffe on the neck.

It would be restorative to the medical profession if instead of taking itself seriously, it took the patients that way.

When composer Tom Whitman first told me, after reading my short story " 'The Black Swan' Revisited," that he found it operatic in tone, I was pleased. And not a little worried. I have long been a lover of opera, mostly Italian with a little French thrown in and a large heaping of Mozart. A while later he informed me that he planned to compose an opera based on that story, which I had adapted from a novella by Thomas Mann, *Die Betrogene*, "The Deceived Woman." Now I was really worried. The story of Rosalie von Tummler is histrionic, if not downright melodramatic. There is a single powerful theme—that death comes to her in the guise of love. The deception is not cruel but merciful. Everything in the story, and in an opera based upon it, must contribute to the presentation of this theme. The libretto must be pared down to utter simplicity for the impact to be given through that most evocative and stirring instrument, the human voice.

Libretto means "little book," and there are few littler books than the text of an opera. No one I know has ever read a libretto for pleasure alone. An exception is Maurice Maeterlinck's *Pelléas et Mélisande*, every word of which was set to music by Debussy. Another is Ralph Vaughan Williams's *Riders to the Sea*, in which he has been faithful to J. M. Synge's text. A great play is not a great libretto for the reason that it is *not* a little book and doesn't need music to enhance it. In the simplification necessary for opera, the literature upon which it is based may disappear—style, masterful use of language, the color and texture of the writer's mind (in this case that of Thomas Mann)—and all that is left is a simple plot and the bold depiction of characters. All opera is melodrama in that it appeals not just to the intellect but to the heart as well. Melodrama is nothing if not fair. Gilda is the corrupt Rigoletto's soul exteriorized. This is made manifest when she sings "Caro nome." At that moment she becomes insubstantial. It is expected that the cruel jester will pay the ultimate price, the loss of his soul, for his debased life at court. Likewise, Rosalie is given the illusion of youth and love but must pay for it with her life.

In many operas derived from stories, most of the characters are lost. In rewriting Mann's novella, I myself dispensed with the younger brother of Anna (Rosalie's daughter), and I amalgamated three doctors into one,

Doctor Hahn, a former lover of Rosalie's. The handsome Ken, who in Mann was a device and rather a stick figure or foil for Rosalie's passion, I turned into a complicated young man with problems of his own. My story becomes a kind of domestic triangle with Ken, Anna, and Rosalie reacting among themselves. Whitman's operatic version has dismissed Doctor Hahn from the premises and pares down the action to a minimum, relying on music and voice to carry the day.

But there is another element in "The Black Swan" that descends from Mann to me and is carried through into the opera. That is the mystical otherworldliness of the theme. That a woman under the spell of a powerful and hopeless passion should grow progressively younger as the drama advances, and that she and her daughter should both be deceived by this, would be, if true, a violation of the natural order of things. However, it is precisely her surrender to this "supernatural" phenomenon—the return of her youthful appearance, which she sees with her own eyes, after all—that propels the plot of the opera. In the hands of a great actress, Rosalie can fool the audience, no matter how modern and sophisticated, into believing the impossible. She seduces the audience into her own deception. I have seen that happen, so that when the terrible truth is revealed late in the play—that the return of her youthful appearance is due, in fact, to cancer—there is a gasp of dismay in the theater.

Opera brings us directly into the world of archetypes, and this is done by music alone. As E. T. A. Hoffmann put it: "The lyre of Orpheus opens the door of the Underworld," and the Underworld is the home of archetypes: inherited, primitive ideas that are most easily recognized in mythology. We respond to Rosalie's deception, her sojourn in the supernatural, because it awakens hidden dreams and desires that lie deep inside us. The composer of opera speaks to us from the archetypal roots of his own psyche.

With age I am become the most suggestible of readers. I have only to settle into a story when I fall into a strange blend of reverie and restlessness. Then it is that I remember and imagine, or both—I can no longer say for sure. For example, reading Anzia Yezierska's novel *Bread Givers* has awakened a memory long submerged. Or at least I assume it's a memory. Trouble is, if *I* don't know, who is there alive who can tell me?

I was ten years old. It was summer in Toronto, the same summer Uncle Max took me to see the Masked Marvel wrestle against the Angel at the Maple Leaf Gardens, an incident recounted in *Confessions of a Knife*. One Sunday we went on a picnic to an island in Lake Ontario. It was crowded with Jews from the city. There was a good deal of hawking of cooked foods and *tchatchkes*. The older men were bearded and wore yarmulkes. I remember the hilarity that prevailed and the often cruel ethnic humor. Then a man with an accordion and a woman stood in a small clearing. What a contrast between the two performers: she a heavy woman with bleached blond hair wearing every color, he a skinny *krotzer*. Aunt Sarah explained to me that this woman, a great favorite, was a widow who had lost her son to T.B. After a brief flourish and cadenza from the accordion, she began in a voice that was at once subdued, sobbing, and eloquent. "Sun, thou shin'st on everyone else, only not on me . . ." Well—it sounds better in Yiddish. It certainly rang home to the crowd, for the women began weeping, and even some of the men were wiping away moisture with the backs of their horny hands. As she sang these songs about love lost, premature death, and life in the shtetl, it seemed to me that *it was the very sadness* the people enjoyed, and that they were having a *laybedickeh tag*—a wonderful time. When she had eaten out everyone's heart, she nodded to the accordionist and broke loose with "Auf'en pripachickl brent a firel, in shteeb bist hayss." Soon the whole crowd was singing. This was followed by comic numbers with lewd lyrics that sent everybody bellowing and shrieking, Aunt Sarah included. How do I know the lyrics were lewd? Because I asked Aunt Sarah what could be so amusing. "None of your business," she sputtered in the dyspnea of laughter.

Did this really happen, and had I forgotten that day for so long? Real or imagined, I have Anzia Yezierska to thank for it.

શ્ર

M. arrived precisely on her birthday. The gift I gave her was one day of my life, in which I was to edit the manuscript of her book, which purports to tell the story of her illness, confinement, and the cruel way in which she was treated by the psychiatrists. Although she has been ill (manic-depression) for twenty-five years, she still denies that she is sick, though not always. M. is devoid of literary talent. The manuscript is execrable. Unable to injure this pathetic woman, I line-edited all fifteen chapters while she took notes. Like all loonies, she is utterly self-absorbed, wants to show her achievements, and exults over them like a child. Once again I informed her that we could *not* be lovers and that I was extremely married. The following morning I went to her hotel to say good-bye.

"How long have you been sick?"

"I'm *not* sick. Stop saying that. It makes me feel bad. When I was a girl in Hong Kong my mother threw me into the nut house. It was unjust. Don't worry, I'm calm."

The sight of this twitching, grimacing, monkey-faced woman with an anxiously furrowed brow, given to sudden outbursts of profanity ("Shit!" "Fuck!") has the effect of breaking down my resistance (my flaw).

"When can I come to see you again?"

"You may *not* come back."

"But why?"

"Because you have fallen in love with me, that's why. To let you return would be cruel and stupid. It would only exacerbate your pain."

"Can I walk you to the library?"

"Okay."

"Will you buy me an orange juice?"

"Sure."

At the Educated Burgher I watch her drink the juice. When she is finished, I stand and go out of the restaurant. A brief but fatal backward glance turns my blood to brine. The poor slumped and desolate woman whom I have just banished.

The perpetual malpractice of the computer has put me in a bituminous mood. This has not been lightened by the prospect of a daily e-mail message from M. The two I've received average seven thousand words. *Why* did I give her my e-mail address?

Met one of my other loonies on the street, his nostrils dribbling like a horse with glanders. He wore a frayed and faded necktie of incalculable age. The history of its stains would make a novel. I gave him ten bucks.

The internist, like the shaman, heals the sick mainly by means of language, potions, and charms. The surgeon does it by cutting into the body. The magician and shaman, that is to say the internist, maintains the natural distance between the sick and the one who tends them. The surgeon does the opposite. He penetrates into the body in order to solve the problems of the flesh. At the decisive moment, the surgeon, unlike the internist, does not go face to face with the patient. He covers him up except for the route of entry. It is a fundamental difference between the two healers.

Most deeply "religious" people prefer their mysticism to be thickened with pomp, ceremony, music, procession, and incense. Otherwise it gets to be too cloudy to grab hold of.

Letter from Peter Josyph asking for a word to mean *contempt for dogs*. I gave him *canimosity*. As for my own personal abhorrence, it is the cat. Spare me any such *felicity*.

Thomas Eakins's *The Veteran* is my favorite portrait in the world. It's silly and amateurish to have a favorite portrait, but in *The Veteran*, Eakins has painted more than the face of his model, George Reynolds. Here the face is the echo of Reynolds's soul. There is between subject and painter a feeling that cannot be faked. Whatever it was that Thomas Eakins may have felt for George Reynolds, there are few secrets that art cannot reveal. A portrait is what the artist sees. It is also what he thinks of what he sees. Eakins painted his *Veteran* with a tenderness that suggests a lover.

Time was when art had a ritual or cult value. It was an instrument of magic, and as such remained largely hidden from the public and was exhibited only on special occasions. This still happens when, on the feast days of saints, the relic or statue of the saint is carried in procession through the streets. Nowadays art has an exhibition value: it is meant *to be shown.* Only in portraiture does the cult of remembrance of the dead persist. That is what gives so many portraits an aura of melancholy and incomparable beauty.

In an epistolary fit I wrote twelve letters. In addition to the usual correspondents, I wrote to a reader shocked at my acknowledged atheism: "Even without religion, life is worth living."

I think now that I never had any faith. That appalling Jehovah, the God of Vengeance, who demanded the sacrifice of living animals and who punished Lot's wife for turning around—among his numberless other cruelties—was never mine. Then along came Jesus Christ, who turned himself into a human sacrifice and instructed his followers to eat his body and drink his blood "in remembrance of me." What I did like about the holy cannibalism was the way it was phrased in Latin: *hic est enim Calix Sanguinis mei.* Mysterious, yes, and luscious; but not for me the basis of belief, and savage enough to suit a religion that has caused so much other blood to be shed in its name. And yet, ironically, I spend an inordinate amount of time chewing the cud of Judaism and Christianity. Two thousand years ago I'd have been drawing fish on the walls of the Catacombs.

The novels of Sir Walter Scott and Balzac are no longer readable by me. I haven't the patience to swim through lake after lake of ponderous talk or detailed description in search of a single passage of beauty and truth. They are monotonous and stupefying in a way that painting and sculpture are not. A single glance at a painting can capture the imagination or dismiss the artist as inconsequential.

The painting that lies next to my heart is not *The Veteran* by Eakins or the *Saint Peter* of Juseppe de Ribera. No, it is a picture by Jacob Walker, dated 1814 and done during a certain art class. The painting is a watercolor bouquet of red nasturtiums, pink poppies, and a single blue iris. It hangs directly over the toilet in my first-floor bathroom. It is that blue iris that has helped me to pee all during this past decade of prostatic hypertrophy. It seems that some bladders respond to the color blue by contracting. All thanks to Jacob Walker, my idea of a urologist.

Tomorrow I deliver a sermon at a Unitarian church. I looked up the word *sermon*, a "religious discourse delivered by a clergyman as part of a worship service, or a lecture on conduct or duty." Considering that I am of no religious persuasion—if forced to bow down I would choose to worship fire—and considering that I am chock-full of vice, love sin, and detest abstractions such as "duty" and "conduct," I am ill-equipped to step up to an altar. But if anywhere, a Unitarian church. The first hurdle will be *finding* the church.

This morning at eight o'clock, M. phoned (against the rules). I allowed her to talk for thirty minutes and offered it up. She sang two endless songs over the phone: "Blowing in the Wind" and "Puff, the Magic Dragon." I was touched by her thin quavering childish voice, her need to show off for me, also like a child. She will use any excuse to approach me. "Happy Halloween!" she cried. I believe she has slipped some, is doing a lot of crying, pondering death by suicide. The need is a bottomless pit. I give in for a while, then, as gently as I can, extricate myself and hang up while she is still talking.

Watched a woman eating at the Educated Burgher. She is not one of the regulars. First she took a tiny bite of sandwich, then she covered her mouth with a napkin as if mastication were an act best committed in privacy.

In the daily letter from M. she informs me that she is in love with one Robert, a man from China, that she is hoping to marry him, and that, should he predecease her, she will come to New Haven so that I can assist her suicide. I reiterated her unsuitability for marriage and told her it was better to go on being friends. I am interfering in another's life, but I cannot keep silent on the eve of what I perceive as the deluge. Who and what is this Robert who will enter into a relationship with such a profoundly sick woman? This is the event that could send her tumbling into the abyss again.

Diagnosed Janet as having an impacted lower left ureteral stone with some pyelonephrosis. A week ago she'd had an endometrial biopsy for abnormal bleeding. After a week of having been deceived by the coincidence, it became clear that the one had nothing to do with the other. Poor woman, prowling the house, unable to sit still, like the shark that must keep in constant motion lest it sink and drown. I brought her to her gynecologist and handed him the diagnosis. She is scheduled for ureterolithotomy tomorrow. It does no good to one's self-esteem to be a coward and to have such an absurdly brave wife. It is only *one* of my shortcomings. I am good for nothing but writing, am alive only when writing—I am a man-shaped heap of commas, exclamation points, lyric apostrophes, and metaphors.

Spent the day at Saint Raphael's Hospital, waiting. It seems that the truck bearing the laser (Sun God) from Boston to New Haven had broken down en route. Another laser was requested from New Milford. The surgery scheduled for 8:30 began at 3:30. It was then that the Sun God and Our God Which Art in Heaven (urologist) conjoined to perform a ureterolithotomy. While my nerves were by now quite frayed, Janet accepted the delay with a horrible calm and sweetness. She just sat there receiving the apologies of one and all, visited by any number of doctors and nurses, gossiped with her new colleagues, with whom she exchanged all the intimacies of the flesh: hemorrhoids, carpal-tunnel syndrome, ureteral stone, and so on—and read a novel! Nothing in her entire life becomes her like the prospect of leaving it. In the interstices of this schedule, we behaved toward each other like perfect strangers, with immense consideration, affection, and numerous expressions of mutual concern.

The surgery went well. God informed me that he has been reading *Down from Troy*. I brought Janet home in the dark, gave her noodle soup and a sweet muffin with cream cheese. For me, though, the road wound uphill all the way. Nor was my mood elevated by the squalor of medicine. It is gray, tasteless, commercial, a herding, devoid of wit or intellect. Once again there was the shallowness and narrowness of the doctors. Were they ever my colleagues? All my life I have so much wanted to belong to whatever the prevailing society—athletes, roommates, fellow surgeons—and I went so far as to throttle what was indecent and wild in me. It wasn't any use: I could never be one of them. It was decades before I discovered that what was indecent and wild in me was the source of my art. But these surgeons can do what I can no longer do. I must pay my respects to that. Yet one and all spoke to me of retirement, and not a single one expressed joy in his practice. Then again, there were the lovely, warm, and kindly nurses. No wonder I have always loved them.

As Janet's recovery progresses, we are once again living in a state of sinister coziness. This morning, a lovely autumn Sunday, we walked around Mill River in the park. A pair of swans and their reflections, a family of mallards, the belted kingfisher all in a blizzard of leaves, the entire park like the burnished bronze of Achilles' shield.

My poor M.! She is again adrift in the squalls of her madness. In one day I received a phone call, a tape, and a long letter. I simply had to write saying not to phone again and to write no more than once a month. I tried to explain as gently as possible that she was infringing on my life to the point of severe discomfort. The fact is that she needs nothing from me but the chance to ventilate, sing songs, build castles in the air. I am not allowed to hang up the phone, I am asked if I've heard each tape, and why haven't I answered her letters? It can't go on. And yet I am well aware of her pain. I mailed the letter and felt awful all day.

Walked home at dusk. Inside the Bamboo Forest, night had already installed itself. I trudged through a thick layer of fallen leaves that betrayed every footstep. Suddenly I went "zero at the bone." Just ahead on the path, an animal—fat, with a long skinny tail and a whitish snout.

There it crouched, immobile, its glittering eye! Would it spring? Not a raccoon, nor a rat, nor a squirrel. I took one step backward, then another, whereupon the opossum scurried out of sight.

※

I am one loony less. It had to happen. N. arrived at the library, calling out my name, wilder than usual. I carried out the secretarial tasks involving numbers that trigger his compulsion, a chore that is nothing less than torture for me. After which he went on the attack.

"You are ruthless. You are a phony liberal. You are sympathetic to homosexuals who deserve no sympathy, nor do the handicapped." His hatred of gays is rabid. Then a threat that if I mention him in my diary, he will . . . but he doesn't complete the threat. He has worked himself into a rage. I shook him off at last, went home and phoned him.

"You're fired!" I said. The expected shrieks of fury, self-defense, no speck of self-doubt: he is never at fault. Then the usual psychoanalytic dissection of my mind.

"It's my madness that offends you, isn't it?"

"Your madness not at all. It is the only part of you I can abide. Besides, for years it has provided me with the opportunity to do good works." I regret having said that. On and on he railed, but *en fin* it was "Good-bye and good luck." Incision and drainage, the best way to treat an abscess. It brings relief but no pleasure. The throbbing of pus under pressure is gone, but there remains the sharp sting of the blade. As Carlyle said of listening to Coleridge: "To sit as a passive bucket and be pumped into, whether you consent or not, can in the long-run be exhilarating to no creature." But even as I hung up the phone there came a wave of remorse. I want my loony back.

※

December always grays me up. Skin, hair, eyes, and mood—all are overcast. I feel I am once again in the balaclava of old, itching to rip it off. The trip to France looms, when Janet leaves with Becky on the 25th. I follow three days later. I long to see Jon, but I quail at the journey. The days till then will be spent fishing among books in the library, half hoping that none will be caught. The casting is all.

Went out back to see what's being done to the Taft Mansion. It wears a scaffold of planks, slats, and ladders. A human being actually stepped out of an upstairs window, waved to me, then went back inside. After decades of neglect, Yale has been pressured into "preserving" it. The immediate neighborhood will surely take on airs. We will not be able to sit in the garden in our jammies or pick blackberries on the Yale property.

Some days ago, right here in our neighborhood, a twenty-one-year-old Yale senior, a woman, was murdered, her body left lying in the street. I said *woman* but I mean *girl*, as in granddaughter. Death at that age returns one to childhood, feminism notwithstanding. The event has plunged the entire university and the neighborhood into despondency. We slouch around close to tears. There are no clues, no suspects—the trail is already cold. The *New Haven Register* disgraced itself with a recent headline: "Cops Grill Yale Teacher." The man was her political science professor and thesis advisor. There never was any notion that he was the killer, but there was his photograph on the front page. It is typical of the irresponsible journalism that prevails: news by insinuation and innuendo, the word *grill* dripped lewdly onto the page with all its implications of guilt. Now that he is no longer a suspect, will the *Register* print an apology? Oh, yes, it surely will . . .

Went to print out the ultimate version of "A Fairy Tale" (ultimate for now). The owner of the store is a woman with what might be called a strong personality. Well into her middle age, she has black hair and eyes and is much too short and tubby to wear the louche miniskirts she favors. She is a passionate talker, each word delivered emphatically as if it were of prime importance. In reply to my "How are you," which I did not think of as a question, she embarked upon a long lamentation over her daughter who, at fifteen, has an eating disorder which rollicks her weight from 80 to 140 pounds. She is presently at the upper end of the scale, can't "fit into her pants," is "bloated around the middle," and is woeful. Mother raged at the pediatricians who insinuate that the affliction is all in her daughter's head. "What do you think?" she asked.

I recognized this as a real question, requiring an answer right that second. There was a note of *or else* in her voice. I tried to coin a few words of sympathy, but could think of nothing to say. Whereupon I received this salvo: "If *you* got out of bed in the morning feeling bloated and couldn't get into *your* pants, how would *you* feel if *some doctor* told you it was *all in your head*?" The woman grew *oppugnant*, as Odysseus said of his fellow Greeks outside the walls of Troy. Her breathing was angry. One felt buffeted by her consonants, especially her *p*'s, *t*'s and *b*'s. She was glaring—not at me, but at doctors in general. Then she put a Life Saver in her mouth, where it clicked against her teeth, a good sign that the end was near. I waited to see if there would be more to the eruption or whether she had been sated. "A dollar sixty," she said in a transactional tone of voice.

Now while I love to overhear such private outpourings, I am not fond of having them told to my face. Besides, I only went there to copy "A Fairy Tale." When I related all of this to my daughter Gretchen, she said that I should never, never say *How are you* to anyone. " 'Yo!' doesn't expect to be answered," she said.

Listened to a tape of my talk on *The Dying Centaur* at Cooper Union, and cringed at the sound of my voice, which is thin, high-pitched, reedy, and effeminate. On laryngeal grounds alone I should renounce all rights to the podium forever. I mentioned this to one of the library workers, who told me that nobody likes his own voice, but I suspect she meant to bolster. From there I adjourned to the L & B (Linonia and Brothers) Reading Room at Sterling, where every day I am awakened from my nap by a vacuum cleaner. It is pushed and pulled all day by an elderly black lady with kyphoscoliosis whose sole responsibility must be to keep this vast room tidy. She wears a Yale blue smock, baggy black pants, sneakers, plastic gloves, an old circular straw hat, and horn-rimmed glasses. For jewelry, earrings of bright metal and a broad copper bracelet. A face mask dangles at her neck. Once in a while she raises it to her mouth for a few breaths. Hers is the sweetest smile in all the Ivy League. Her religious faith is absolute and deep.

"I don't have to worry about anything, because I know Jesus will take care of me." Then, after a moment of silence: "They's some folks over the Law Library who don't believe in God. They say they's one of those whatchacallit."

"Atheists."

"Atheists. Do you believe in God? If you don't, I don't want to talk to you."

"Oh yes, I do."

"Well then, that's all right."

The only other occupant of the L & B is a beautiful young graduate student, also trying to sleep. If this were an old movie and I were Cary Grant, I'd slip the cleaning lady a five and nod her off the premises. The noise of the vacuum cleaner grows fainter.

"Shouldn't we talk?" I say to the girl.

She opens her eyes and brings me into focus.

"After all, we *have* been sleeping together."

Her posture stiffens.

"In a manner of speaking."

I am using the baritone tremolo which has served me well in social situations.

"I mean, we *were* both asleep in the same room, weren't we?"

A tiny smile plays about her lips.

"I suppose it's worth a conversation," she says in the manner of Carole Lombard.

Can't a day go by without my shedding daydreams?

Yesterday I made my habitual Sunday morning ascent of East Rock. Not a single jogger or dog walker. *Tout seul*, I imagine because of the murder, still unsolved. In the afternoon I went to row at the gym. The Shower Room is a long rectangular space with five shower heads on either long side and no partitions. Two men, youngish, good-looking, opposite each other, sending messages, at first tentative, furtive—something more than a glance, less than a stare—then reckless, a lazy full-front slow-motion lathering of the genitalia and the erection of one. A burning gaze was exchanged that asked the unmistakable question and gave the unequivocal answer. Suddenly it seemed an aperture had appeared through which one would pass to join the other, as when two parts of a spaceship have docked and an astronaut floats through to greet a new arrival. The necessity to keep looking at them . . . the inability to pull my eyes away from an intimacy I had no right to see . . . the hasty departure of the pair from the Shower Room . . . the headlong, weightless hurtle into orbit . . . the Shower Room strangely quiet in the wake of their assignation.

Met with Nick Frankfort, undergraduate artist and writer, who had asked to show me his work. The boy himself is his greatest work of art: intelligent, serious, mature, handsome. Courteous without being deferential, and with the self-confident ease of an athlete (he's on the university rowing team). He prepared for this meeting with great care, having selected a wide assortment of his work to show me. The pen-and-ink drawings are of dinosaur skeletons. They are intricate, precise, and delicate. His oils too are subtle and surprising. The three prose pieces are rather raw, as one might expect, as he has done little writing as yet. Still there is something that is worthy of developing. We talked about the "writing life" and the wisdom of trying to marry both his interests, writing and painting. I also met with Stuart Davenport, a graduate student writing on a historical aspect of Christianity and politics. Refined, modest, hardworking, and deeply religious, he is tall and blond, with a harmonious body devoid of awkwardness. Stuart too dreams of a life in writing. It appears that I have come to embody Possibility for a number of authors-to-be. A high purpose, indeed, and one for which I'm grateful, if only for the chance to meet so many young people on the brink.

Asked how I remembered my childhood so vividly, I told them that I reinvented rather than recalled it. Besides, the past looms larger and larger right up to the moment of death. I said, too, that I was one of those hateful children who sit and watch and listen. Such a child doesn't smile, doesn't speak, only observes, his pupils dilating and constricting, his breath gone shallow and quick or slow, or stopping, even, in the receptacular act. He is always partly in the shadow, or gives that effect. He is the sort of child you see when you look over your shoulder to see if anyone is there. No need to wonder: *he is*. And your voice lowers so as not to be overheard. No use to tell this child to go outdoors and play ball. He clings to the indoors as he clings to his privacy. It is there that he finds his calling. Attic and cellar know him. He is a daemon.

I was asked also what I meant by the prophetic nature of certain writings: fairy tales and myths. I believe it lies in their timelessness. It doesn't matter when the story takes place, whether past, present, or future, any more than it matters to any human purpose that the light of the stars takes so long to reach the earth. To us who gaze up at the "shining gears of Heaven," there is that which was long ago, is now, and shall be, all at the same moment. Doubtless there will arise a swarm of *vespatious* astronomers to dispute this darling notion, but it is true that in a myth or a fairy tale, prophecy and destiny come together. The fulfillment of a story lies in its being read. That is its destiny. If *Thou shalt be read* is the prophecy made by the author to his story, then the writer who puts himself *inside* a story will read it and discover his own fate. By the author writing in the historical present tense, past and present become coeval. Presumably this can apply to the future as well. In "A Fairy Tale" the doctor rediscovers, through a mauve dove, the passion of an old love. It is more than a memory, for he experiences anew the ancient physical passion at the touch of the dove. It is a passion that took place long ago and is taking place now.

I am standing at the corner of Wall and College streets waiting for the shuttle bus. A car pulls over to the curb. The driver is a comely woman of about forty with a child in the front seat. The window is rolled down.

"Can you tell me where I can find Beecher Street?"

"There is no Beecher Street."

"Oh but there is, and I need to find it."

"I have been at Yale for forty-five years, and one of the things I have learned is that there is no Beecher Street."

"I'm trying to find the Department of Religious Studies."

"Do you mean the Divinity School?"

"No, I'm *at* the Divinity School myself."

"Sorry, I have no idea where Beecher Street is."

"You look so handsome!"

"___!"

Sitting on the shuttle in my blue blazer, white woolen scarf, peak cap, and corduroy pants, I had to agree with her.

The other day at the library, a woman approaches the table where I am writing.

"They tell me you are a doctor."

She speaks in a lilting genteel voice. She tells me the story of her daughter's ten-year struggle with a rare form of lupus. Did I by any chance know her doctor? I did. When the daughter passed away, she undertook to rear her grandson and see him well educated. He is presently a senior at Yale, where she works as a cleaning lady. I am drawn into her situation. There is not a speck of self-pity or gloom. She is merely telling her story. A typical day at the library.

Janet is off to France. I phoned a friend I hadn't seen in fifteen years to wish him season's greetings. We had been together in a sporadic, opportunistic way, as men at a university often are. After some months my interest dwindled to mere curiosity, and I saw him more out of habit than anything else. He was always drunk when I arrived, the apartment full of smoke, his face an open wound of loneliness that I could have fallen into. I would stay, listening to his monologue, until he staggered and fell. I would drag him to the bed, then let myself out. I suppose the reason I kept on with it was that naked loneliness on his face. He is not unintelligent. A Yale graduate and a voracious reader, he has worked at the university for fourteen years. He is happy in his job and has managed to keep the drinking and smoking apart from it. I had run into him on the street and thought, Well, why not? And so I phoned.

He answered the door in shorts and T-shirt, cigarette in hand, the air blue behind him. That familiar loose-lipped grin. Drunk, I decided, and I saw on the desk, alongside an open book, a glass of white wine with the bottle nearby. Ten cigarette butts in an ashtray. The one room is quite beautifully decorated and well kept. The bed wears an Indian bedspread, his pictures are on the walls, there is a small balcony with a view of Long Island Sound. For the next two hours he drank and smoked, smoked and drank. And talked. Hardly what you'd call a conversation. I was but the most welcome receptacle into which he poured his thoughts on numerous issues. I decided not to wait for the collapse and stood to leave.

"Don't go yet! *Please* don't go. Don't leave me. Not yet."

Fifteen years later, the same desperation, the same fear of being alone.

"Good-bye," I announced to let him know I wouldn't be coming again. Once in my car, a wave of pity and, yes, guilt. I could have stayed another hour and left after he had passed out. Along the streets, men gesticulating at me, waving their arms. What could it mean? Did they know something about me? Not until I reached the bottom of my drive-way did I awake to the fact that I hadn't turned on the headlights.

A day tout seul chez moi. Tried to write, but the words I needed the pen could not limn. Went to the piano for solace, only to find that the notes I sought lay between the keys. Listened to *The Magic Flute*. Two great voices, Sarastro and Papageno. Wrote ten letters, one to a psychologist who is investigating the phenomenon of visual hallucinations in the blind. What he calls "phantom vision," to relate it to phantom limb. Aparrently these are quite common, varied, and interesting both to the one who experiences them and to the psychologist. They are multicolored and consist of many different moving images. Some are dramatic, religious, or archetypal, others are of mundane objects. One subject experienced the feeling that the chair in which he was sitting rose into the air and became enveloped with green foliage. There is a tendency to fail to report or to deny these hallucinations so as not to be considered peculiar or crazy. In phantom limb, the missing limb is experienced. It occupies a position in space and can generate sensation such as pain and heat. Auditory halluci-nations have been reported in people with hearing loss. It seems likely that a similar "neuropsychological" mechanism accounts for all of these and provides a sensory-perceptual "fill." Is there some neural network for the "body self" that generates these hallucinations? Some of these hallucinations are threatening, even dangerous, but some can be quite companionable and can give the feeling that one can *actually* see.

This is a fascinating subject which tempts me to write a short story about a blind man who experiences phantom vision to a high degree. The premise will be that there is another life of the body that is being lived at the same time as the one we are aware of, only this second body-life is hidden, subtle, able to be called forth only by the impaired, who can tap into it. Phantom vision would occur only in someone who had gone blind after years of seeing, not in one who was born blind. I must think of this phenomenon and its ramifications. Could this be at the bottom of all the "visitations" of Mary and Jesus? Could Francis of Assisi, Theresa of Avila, and Catherine of Siena have been severely neurotic people who could call upon this second, underlying body-life? Catherine, who was anorexic, would be a likely candidate.

1999

THE RAIN AND WIND OF THE past few days have spent themselves. Now, down from a huge blue sky, flocks of juncos are sown into every clump of bushes the way Shakespeare hung a cuckoo on every tree.

From four in the morning on, the raccoons in heated debate in the garden.

Informed by a Yale undergraduate, one Eli Kintich (let his name live on in infamy), that he has lost the photo of Vladimir Petrov that I lent him during his interview of me. The photo shows a broadly smiling old man, well into his eighties, looking bright, healthy, and alert. In the attached note he reminded me that thirty-seven years earlier I had performed an emergency subtotal gastrectomy on him for massive upper gastrointestinal hemorrhage. It was just short of exsanguination, I remember. I was thrilled to have the photo—now, through the carelessness of youth, lost. Quite cast down about this, mind clouded up. Add to that a letter from M., first in a month, as I have restricted. She spent the past three weeks in hospital again, is quite mad, rattled on about going back to Hong Kong, and about this "fiancé" who is married to someone else.

Took a friend to the Elizabethan Club, where R.V., of ancient Middle Eastern languages—Sumerian, Akkadian, Hittite—introduced to us his colleague, who is gorgeous, young, and blond. I asked if they worked together. No, she is much later, beginning in 600 B.C., while R.V. goes back a few thousand years earlier. We stood around for ten minutes, the two men feasting on her, she casting *schwas* at each of us with deadly aim.

If the practice of medicine teaches anything, it is that the pronoun *we* is not plural, but singular. One fate awaits us.

Caught sight on the street of a shabby old man with uncombed gray hair under a plaid cap, baggy corduroys, a blue-and-white shirt, black vest, and scuffed shoes. It's me! Then came the fever. To Sterling for a sit-down, lurching like a lobster who's missing one claw.

Marvelous review of *The Doctor Stories* in the Galveston, Texas, newspaper by a Dr. Melvyn Schreiber. I'll write to thank him, even though one mustn't, according to the etiquette of criticism. One is hardly immune to such tickling.

Alsace-Lorraine. Son Jon and his wife, Regine, raise their children with infinite patience. There is no speck of mean authority in it. Danny and Emmy squabble like an elderly Mormon couple who had, decades before, been joined for time and eternity in the tabernacle. While they cannot be separated, each must carve out his turf with an electron microscope, dividing up the mitochondria equally. The settlement in which Jon lives consists of several hundred newly constructed houses, each more charmless than the next. It is called La Domaine du Golfe, after the golf course

on the premises. It is a five-mile walk into the main village of La Wantze-
nau for croissants and bread every morning, the time I cherish. By every
plowed field there is a stone crucifix. Sunday church services are attended
by a handful of the elderly. One wonders if the rest are rosary chewers in
time of need (*macheux de capelots*). I am trying not to fall into a *rouge-noir*
(melancholy). It is too easy to do here. As for religion, one doesn't need
the Garden of Gethsemane when one has La Domaine du Golfe.

All this French—I have little resistance to it here.

Home. At Last. I remain an adjunct to my upper respiratory tract. Three
weeks of cough, coryza, and (doubtless) consumption, along with the
whole panoply of *rrheas*—dia, rhino, broncho, everything but gono—
have shrunk the rest of the corpus down to filaments and beads. Even so,
the tic of writing persists. The pen jerks words out of the empty air and
flips them down onto the page where they lie quivering. So writeth the old
bale of straw, cinched at the middle with a kind of abject anatomical
sagaciousness above and below. Every day another button commits suicide, a seam opens itself, a lining hangs out in plain sight. No pocket but is
stuffed with Kleenex, toilet paper, napkins . . . whatever might stanch the
tide. At the Law School cafeteria, carrying coffee and a biscuit to a table, I
had a sudden jerk and spilled it all. A workman brought napkins and
mopped me and the floor. I began again, only to drop a knife this time.
Another workman rushed up. "Here, let me get that for you." And before
I could protest he had picked up the knife and taken away my tray.
Imagine! From professor of surgery I have become a stumbler and a
spiller, a sad old sheep whose paraphernalia and food keep raining down.
Drooling is next. And now look! A leaky pen. A big blue stain on my
shirt, and blue up to the second interphalangeal joint of my index finger.

Led to the piano in accordance with a will other than my own (I had not touched it in months), I played all of *Beliebte Meisterstücke auf alte Zeit* with every one of the repeats and da capos. It took three hours and fifteen minutes. With that out of my system I could get on with my journal. Nature has done rather well by me in some ways, but I am not organized for the piano.

I might as well stop reading *Troilus and Cressida*, as I've decided against giving the seminar on Shakespeare and *A Month in the Country*. It would have been a new challenge for me, but the fee to take it is $250, for which the students deserve a professional theater maven, not a Teaching Assistant who reads the plays for the first time and has never seen them produced. I am an impostor, yes, but not of that magnitude. Also I am offended by the young administrator, a woman who is officious and disrespectful. I am feeling guilt over backing out of it but also a sense of relief at having shucked a deadline as well as the feeling of being a poseur.

Read in the *New York Times* of some New York City policemen who have advanced degrees in classics and English literature. Doubtless they could not find teaching jobs and are now cops. The very best reason to write another book would be if one of these young officers were to carry it in his breast pocket. Now say that he catches a perpetrator in an act of burglary. The criminal shoots him at point-blank range but he isn't hurt, as the book—*Mortal Lessons*, for instance—deflected the bullet. That alone would be worthy of the National Book Award.

I am sitting in the computer cluster at the library. Next to me, a man who grunts passionately and snuffles every few seconds even as he types. His is a soft grunt and so is not terribly distracting. Nevertheless he is isolated by his affliction, set aside by the rest who are mostly students. They take pains not to notice him and not to embarrass him. He appears to be about my age, is slender, small, and nice looking. While I have not heard him speak, I have the impression that he is foreign, a European. I have diagnosed him as Obsessive Compulsive Disorder, of the Tourette variation, only the outburst constricted down to the grunting and snuffling.

The city streets are flooded from the great gray rain that came right after the snowfall. Whereupon Jack Frost pulled the carpet out from under and the whole mess froze. Now for two days it has been melting. My carrel at Cross Campus Library, which abuts the glass wall of the well outside, is flooded, the carpet entirely submerged and gone from gray to a distinctly feculent brown. Only one manuscript was damaged. I am trying to dry it out page by page. And all the while spread my wings like a waterlogged anhinga.

At eleven in the morning, awakened by a security guard in the library.

"You got the whole place to yourself, Doc."

I looked around and saw that it was so.

"Rainin' good outside. Keep it up four or five hours."

With that report he left to make his rounds. It occurs to me that the security guards have made it up among themselves to wake me whenever I'm seen napping, just to make sure I haven't died. Perhaps I *shall* die here. A book will slip from my hand to the floor. No one will notice; a hundred books slip so each afternoon in sleep. I shall have slumped forward with my head resting on the desk, again as in sleep, half-hidden behind the partitions of the cubicle. I shouldn't want to upset the students. Best to remain undiscovered till after closing time. The security guard would discover the corpse. He would have shaken it by a shoulder, called out to it, "Come on now, professor, wake up! You've got yourself locked in. Wake up!" A certain heaviness, a settled look would give it away and the "removal" would be set in motion. A fitting and quiet exitus, all the drama concealed inside the body—a clot flung lungward, perhaps; a ruptured aorta; some bleeding into the brain. Later it would be consolatory to my next of kin: "He died where he wrote, while in the very act of writing. Look! in the middle of a word, even, he stopped. What word was it? *Aqualune* (moonlight on the water)? One of his made-ups." It's as happy as death can arrange itself to be.

The dregs of the flu still herewithin (points to sinuses, chest, throat), but am loitering back along the road to Salubria. Today's chief complaint is thirst, as if Pantagruel has me by the throat. I reached for a book to read at three in the morning. Turned out to be mine: *Taking the World in for Repairs*. It is, I think, one of my better fooleries, although stuffed with *metaphors extracted out of the claustral kettle*, as Friar John says in Rabelais.

Janet and I may be the only two adults in New Haven who have not watched a bit of Bill Clinton's impeachment trial in either the House or the Senate. The very sight of all those suited-up hypocrites would give me a relapse.

News that L.Y. has been diagnosed as having lymphoma. Several months ago he'd asked me to feel a lump in his groin. Non-tender, not stony hard. No fungal or other infection of the foot. Felt it again a week later—unchanged, although L.Y. said that he thought it smaller. I told him to see his doctor. He did, had a normal blood count, felt well, and was advised to watch further. Now here he is having begun his first teaching job, bought a house, and with four children, one an infant. This will call upon all of his sacred obedience and acceptance. I'm quite cast down by this, though buoyed a bit by the cure rates in some forms of lymphoma. Depends, I gather, upon the cell type. Who knows? We squirm, but Fate has her way with us. I wrote to let him know the latest pronouncement of his co-religionist Reverend Jerry Falwell, who wants everyone to know that the Antichrist is abroad and that he is a male Jew. More than once in our religious discussions, I suggested to L.Y. that I might be the A.-C. Not that I'm campaigning for the seat, mind you. But I daresay, L.Y. is not up for tweaking right now.

❧

What it takes for two people to live together in marital harmony is repression. From wedding day on, you must snuff out a good part of the energy, lust, and adventure that swept you to this point in life. So slowly and insidiously does this self-discipline become the modus vivendi that you do not even notice when you have stopped having your own thoughts and ideas. You have already slipped into the marital "we," as in "We vote Democratic," or "As for abortion, we are pro-choice," or "We saw the play and did not find it amusing." In the early years of marriage, fueled by the ardor of youth, such plurality can be mistaken for the *nous d'amour* rather than what it is—the onset of a vegetable state of mind that sets in after about five years.

Still, there are those rare moments of clarity such as happened the other day. Janet and I were sitting in the garden in which the daylilies were blooming and dying on the same day, as is their wont.

"Only a single day of life," she lamented, "it's hardly worth planting them." All at once, much as enlightenment came to Buddha, so was I struck by a shaft of it.

"Not at all," I replied, "that is precisely why they are worth planting. It is in the brevity of the daylily where lies its melancholy charm." Now we can both settle in for another decade of repression.

Just plain sick. Not so as to die but to prevent working, which is a temporary form of the same thing. Yesterday I crawled to the Music Library, asked to hear a Mozart quintet, was sat down in a booth, given earphones, and soon there was Rudolf Serkin et al., after which I felt much better, though liquefied. Ran out of the library and all over the floor.

Tea at the Elizabethan Club with pre-med English major, a guarded sort who looks at you without expression, as though expecting to be hit, but all the while click-click goes the brain and he knows all the answers. His father is an anesthesiologist. The son likes that specialty, as it affords maximum doctor-patient contact! I refrained from pointing out that only one of the two would be awake. Also, he pronounced Proust "Prowst." We were joined by a graduate student in religious history. A devout Christian, very appealing, he said that he was shocked to learn that I was married, had children and grandchildren, but was relieved by news that I am a family man. He had always assumed that I was single.

"You don't wear a ring."

"No, surgeons usually don't—the frequent scrubbing."

I refrained from pointing out that Christ was a bachelor, also Saint Francis of Assisi, and we all know how Saint Paul felt about marriage: "Better to marry than to burn." We are to meet next week when I shall probe for bigotry. I was joined later by another undergraduate who asked if I were the Richard Selzer whose essays and stories he'd read in high school. Quite set up by that. Suddenly, *spento!* And cut it short to head for home.

Sick through and through. Nightsweats requiring two showers and changes of bed. Cough. Fatigue. No such thing as drifting off into the outer reaches of the mind; there is no mind, only a miasma.

To the library, where I sat on a radiator, then to the Lizzie to open the vault that holds the club's Elizabethan treasures (a Friday afternoon ritual). There I was told that Gordon Reid, my beloved doctor, having decided that he was out of date, elected to study all of medicine again by himself and to retake the qualifying examinations. *This is a noble man.*

Letters and gifts from M., who is unable to restrain the barrage. The letters are in an illegible scrawl.

The security guard, a self-styled newspaper reporter, obsessed with the recent murder of a Yale student, speaks of nothing else. She is well on the road to madness and has already co-opted the domain of bad taste. She so much wants the professor under suspicion to be guilty, she is clearly downcast when I offer her nothing but his presumed innocence. "You're his neighbor. Didn't you see anything suspicious?" Her hair is dyed jet black with a gray inch at the crown where it has grown out. She wears it hanging full length and combed down over her face so that she must peer through strands of it. She is drenched with sickish perfume, many brace-lets, necklaces, rings. A study in sexual deprivation of the Linda Tripp genre. And as repellent.

Long lists of questions from Merri Edwards, who is the archivist in Galveston where my papers have been sent. She wants the first or last names of correspondents who long ago flitted in, flapped their wings once or twice, then flitted back out. She is greatly entertained by the quantity of women who have "fallen in love" with me. She speaks of my "adorabil-ity." No use to point to the absurdity of it, that I could be any woman's romantic ideal, all wrists and ribs as I am, except for the little pot belly. I begin to question the wisdom of having let loose this tiger (the Selzer

Archive, not Merri) in Texas. And no matter the zeal and thoroughness of the scholars, there will always be lacunae, which each of them will find it irresistible to fill in according to a variety of preconceptions and prejudices. Then too there is my own "candor," which clouds as much as it clarifies. I haven't the zest to undress my breast and show the wound beneath. What is the point of all this decoding and deciphering if at the end there is just a naked, pale man like any other, emerging from a dim, chilly corridor, shivering and indistinct?

Conducted an expository writing class for Kathy Rodgers. It went rather well, but only rather, I thought. Their text is William Zinsser's *On Writing Well*. I told them it should have been called *On Writing Rather Well*. I regaled them with the ancient story of Zinsser and me debating at Hamden Hall school over accuracy in reporting. I was the doctor in Chapter 1, and I made him change the name under threat of testicular surgery. They asked about gaining the trust of the reader, about my religion, about how to create the *texture* of a piece, about changing careers in mid-life, about . . . all this after a wild night of fever, sweats, and nightmares. But they were so good-looking! I went from the class straight to the gym. The sauna was full of fat men, all so warm and mellow. Coughing and breathless, I could have gratefully fallen into a generous paunch, *any* paunch, for comfort.

Tête-à-tête at the Lizzie with Stuart Davenport, a graduate student writing on the history of Protestantism in America. A deeply religious Christian who is determined to live a life as free of sin as possible, Stuart gives the term *purity* a new luster. His faith is a great crystal escarpment atop which he stands, arms upraised to God. I cannot but marvel at the beauty and power of such a faith. We talked about cynicism. Can one be a cynic and a Christian? I said yes; cynics can be teased out of their negativism. Cynics deplore and deride the very things they would die to achieve or possess. It's a form of self-defense against the feeling of failure or shame. "Besides," I told him, "we cynics are here for the rest of you to forgive."

We talked about writing as a selfish act (Stuart desires to be a writer). Writers, he said, are odd neurotic loners who separate themselves from others in order to watch and observe for their own purposes. Can a writer be fair to a wife and children? I said yes; the writer leaves his lonely table and cleaves unto his family, drawing sustenance from them and giving them love just as any husband and father hopes to do. The problem arises when the spouse has no faith in the writer's talent, decides he is wasting his time and that the family is paying the price for a frivolity. Besides, writing can be pro bono publico. Think of Saint Paul. Stuart confessed to being moody. Ought he to inflict his moods on a wife? "Absolutely," I said. "Find a good Christian woman with whom you can pray and play, and I predict your moodiness will vanish."

This fellow is a sterling specimen of humanity. Like a couple of other devout Christians hereabouts, he finds it easy to be intimate with me, an outsider. He knows that I am not going to be judgmental. I urge him to finish his dissertation, teach at a Christian college, marry and produce good-looking Christian children, and do a little writing. I promised to write to Philip Yancey to introduce him. Philip is the prolific author of many Christian books with titles like *The Jesus I Never Knew*. He is also a fan of mine and once interviewed me for something called *Books and Culture*. Altogether a fine visit, and we are to be friends.

"What shall I call you?" he asked at the door.

"Richard. Nobody calls me Doctor anymore. I'll explain some time."

M. has resumed her bombardment of illegible scrawl, unintelligible tapes of songs that she sings, and packages of Chinese tea. She expects Janet and me to fly to Canada in February for the "publication" of her "book." I had to write yet another of my "brutal" letters, informing her that she had broken the monthly letter rule, and so I would not read any others or listen to the tapes, nor would I drink the tea. I also had to tell her that I'd been sick for a month and have no intention of going anywhere, much less Canada. Then V. phoned and announced that he was going to France for three months, then called back a few minutes later to say that he'd had a heart attack and that, if he dies, I'm to go to his apartment and rescue the manuscript called "God is M' Whispering Wind" before his family destroys it. Next morning, slid under the front door, was a sheet of yellow legal paper: "Dear St. Selz. It's OK I had a small heart attack. Love, V." Thus have I become confessor to loony and saint alike. My only credential is that I am neither.

Further notes from the Ministry. Walked up to Sterling Library, where I was at a table reading. The invader: N., who sat himself on the table.

"What are you reading?"

He doesn't care at all, but it's his opening gambit.

"Gorki. 'Twenty-six Men and a Girl.' "

"Oh, I read that. His best work is the first volume of the autobiography, when he is living with his grandmother."

All this in a loud, unmodulated voice, despite that I have long made it clear that he must whisper so as not to disturb others. There followed a long animated account of his one visit to a gay bath, accompanied by his girlfriend of the moment, whose idea it was. Description of one man buggering another while others watched. Et cetera. No amount of shushing would keep him still. I nodded toward the door and made to get up. At that moment, a young woman turned around and said to us, "Would you please be quiet?" I was mortified and furious. Walked with him to the door.

"You know that you have offended me. I have always tried to keep you from becoming a nuisance to others, and today you have been."

"I got carried away by my story."

"Good-bye."

What makes the mentally ill impossible to tolerate is their utter self-absorption. It is a sea in which they are afloat and tumbling, the medium that they breathe: the Self. They cannot consider the needs of anyone else—it simply doesn't occur to them. Once chastised, yes, there is a moment of insincere apology, but the poor creatures are blind to the least code of social intercourse or friendship. It accounts for their isolation and loneliness. Only a saint (St. Selz) would be willing to enter such a kaleidoscopic association in which his own identity must be surrendered. With the loonies there is no give and take, no waiting your turn. It is all the urgency of the child demanding instant attention. From them I have learned that Reason walks, Madness dances. Reason is blessed with intelligence, Madness is afflicted with ectasy. Or is it the other way around?

Crept to Educated Burgher for a cup of chicken-noodle soup. No sooner seated than V. comes shambling in à la Groucho Marx, unshaven and squinting. He spots me and with a terrible look of triumph sits himself down and leans close.

"Don't sit so close," I tell him. "I have the flu. Been sick for a whole month. A wicked germ."

Instantly his chair slid backward and he was on his feet, muttering to himself.

"I have to go," he called back.

Never was chicken soup so enjoyed. Followed by a delicious pear I'd brought from home.

What with this damn illness added to the usual writer's isolation, I haven't heard a word of the gossip that is the mucilage of peasantry, bourgeoisie, and elite alike. Rather puts one in danger of spinning off into the outer reaches of his own imagination. There is nothing I love better than a good bit of gossip, preferably malicious, but my only contacts this month have been pedagogical or ministerial, and you can't gossip with students or loonies.

Attended a dinner party given by Ruth Lord, who lives around the corner. Large group including a quantity of Yale professors, one of whom insisted on introducing me as "the famous novelist." I was perfectly willing to let it pass and bask in the glow of undeserved praise, but Janet issued the erratum that I had never written a novel and that I was very far from famous. Like the Taj Mahal, she has a way of making one see human glory in contrast to the eternal. Seated at dinner next to Ruth, a woman I both like and admire. She is one of two children of the DuPont who built and lived at Winterthur. She was sent early to private school in New York City and would go home to Delaware for the weekends, always making sure that the chauffeur parked several blocks from the school so that the others would not get wind of her station in life. At Winterthur her governess would be waiting. The weekend would be spent trying to avoid or elude said governess, mostly by horseback riding or other outdoor activities. She has just written a memoir of her adored father, to be published in April by Yale. She did all the research for the book at the "golf cottage," a twenty-six-room house that she still owns on the grounds of the museum. "No one in that family ever threw away a letter," she said. Also, reported Ruth, she never saw her mother without long white gloves. In later life Ruth returned to school and obtained a Ph.D. in child psychology and worked on the staff of the Child Study Center for many years. From her marriage to George Lord, a fine English professor, there issued four children. After dinner I felt the flu taking hold and stood to leave.

"Wasn't the food perfectly awful?" asked Ruth.

"It was."

"And not enough of it," she said.

Ruth is nothing if not candid. A generous, charming woman.

Thinking about circumcision, wondering what's done with the prepuce afterward. Is it merely discarded? If so, the Jews are missing the boat. That would be a waste of the magical potential of that little raglet. There were tribes in central Australia (the Anula and the Warramunga) who buried the foreskin by the side of a pool where bright blue waterlilies grew. The members of these tribes then dined on the stems and roots of the waterlilies. There was a fertilizing virtue ascribed to the buried foreskin and transmitted to the flowers. Among another tribe, the Unmatjera, a boy would carry his foreskin at night into the forest and deposit it in the hollow of a tree known only to himself. This was the tree from which his spirit had emerged at birth, and to which it would return after death. The foreskin secured the future birth and reincarnation of its owner. During the interval between the two incarnations, it lived in the tree. Among the Akikoyo of East Africa, circumcision was combined with a graphic pretense of rebirth enacted by the novice. So the purpose of circumcision, its real meaning, is not just that business about "entering the covenant," but to ensure the rebirth of the circumcised man at some future time. By placing the foreskin within reach of his disembodied spirit, he provides it with the strength and energy to be born again.

This is what comes of browsing in Frazer's *The Golden Bough*. But thirty years ago, in the late sixties or early seventies, I wrote a short story on this theme. It is called "Jungle Becoming." It is one of the first half dozen stories I wrote. I have not seen it since, and can only suppose that it is in the Archive. It would seem that, for each writer, there are certain defining themes. Perhaps circumcision and rebirth is one of mine. Else why this late blooming of interest?

Feeling better today. At lunch and gossiping with the Boys Friendly, I brought up the subject of foreskins, which quickly descended into a sub-Rabelaisian uproar. Gene Waith insisted on describing his circumcision at age thirteen for "adhesions." He had promised that he would never touch his penis again, but broke his word the next day. Asked if I were circumcised, I said that a good writer doesn't tell, he shows. Claude Rawson, our expert on cannibalism, satire, and other arcane matters, said that he'd never met a man who'd "et" foreskin. Suggested to the maitre d' that foreskins on toast be added to Mory's menu for lunch as #4 (after #3, which is half a club sandwich and a bowl of soup). The maitre d' was not amused.

Thinking further about circumcision, or *briss* as it is called in Hebrew: along with trepanning the skull, it must be the oldest surgical operation, performed thousands of years before Jehovah ordered Abraham to circumcise himself at the age of ninety-nine as a token of the covenant between man and his God. Then Abraham circumcised Ishmael and all the men of the household. The very inheritance of the land of Canaan was bound up in this covenant. Failing to do so was to cut yourself off from the body of Israel. The uncircumcised, such as the Philistines, were referred to with contempt. There have been centuries of Talmudic argument about it, such as: *Why hadn't God made man as he wanted him in the first place?* Answer: *It is up to man to perfect himself at the divine command.*

Circumcision is not a sacrament the way baptism is. It is a duty that must be performed on the eighth day of a boy's life. A metal bell-shaped shield is placed over the glans to protect it. The prepuce is drawn up over the bell and a sleeve lowered to fit tightly around the foreskin exterior to the shield. The skin is then cut circumferentially. Until well into the twentieth century the foreskin was further torn down the center as far as the glans, and the *mohel*, or circumcisor, applied suction to the cut with his mouth to draw off the blood and encourage healing. I have circumcised some dozens of babies, but of all the operations that I would now shrink to perform, circumcision stands high, not because of any complexity or risk to the patient, but because of my own displaced castration anxiety. In *Shakespeare and the Jews*, by James Shapiro, in the part which deals with the *Merchant of Venice*, the author advances the interpretation that Shylock's pound of flesh, to be taken from a place near the heart, is a displacement of the ounce of flesh cut off in ritual circumcision. The word *flesh*, he points out, is used to mean *penis* in *Romeo and Juliet* and also, I believe, in the Bible. The *Merchant of Venice* closely follows a source play wherein a pope tells the winner of a wager that, yes, he can cut off a pound of the loser's flesh, but only a pound, not a speck more or less, else he is to forfeit his own life.

In Jeremiah the men of Judah are told to "remove the foreskins of the heart." What could this mean? Later they are told that they should circumcise their ears, that they might be able to heed the warnings of the prophet-scold:

> To whom shall I speak?
> Whom shall I warn, and be heard?
> See! Their ears are uncircumcised
> they cannot give heed. [Jeremiah 6:10]

A few years ago, I was at dalliance with a graduate student who asked me whether I knew that Shakespeare had taken part in translating the Bible into the King James Version. No, I didn't. Well, he had! It seems that Shakespeare was forty-six years old the year the Bible was finished. The task of translation having proved more difficult than expected, those authorized to do so turned to the greatest living writer in their midst for help. With all of the great plays finished and time hanging heavy on his hands, Shakespeare was glad to help. Naturally I berated the arrant liar for his villainy. Whereupon he went to the shelf for the King James.

"Forty-six years old, remember? Turn to Psalm 46 and find the forty-sixth word. What is it?"

I counted.

"Shake," I replied.

"Now count from the end of the psalm (excepting the final *selah*) and tell me the word."

Again I counted.

"Spear," I murmured weakly.

"Typical Shakespearean wordplay," he crowed.

Where do these graduate moles come from?

Interesting conversation with three brilliant young physicists, two still in their twenties. Yoon Bai, one of two Koreans, is the eldest, a husky, authoritative, mild-mannered leader who has a paternal manner with the other two, although he is in his thirties. When I spoke of the pink *jindaleh* (azalea) that covered the hillsides every spring, they were mystified. It seems that there are no barren hillsides; the entire country of Korea has been "developed" down to the last inch. Where, I wondered, are the villages of U-or L-shaped houses with their thatched roofs, verandahs, sliding paper doors, and courtyards for the tethered beasts? Are there no papa-sans with wispy beards and tall horsehair hats? No high-waisted women in turned-up *itiwa* shoes gathering firewood in the hills? Who is fermenting *kimchi* in tall earthen jars? Do farmers plow the paddies behind their red oxen? Does the honey-bucket man come to ladle his product onto the young rice shoots? Or has modern sanitation dispensed with the use of human excrement as fertilizer? Does the white heron, called *hak*, the symbol of long life, still stand motionless in the paddies?

There is none of that. My Korea—and the novel I wrote about it—is as remote as the Middle Ages. I myself am an anachronism, someone who had once traveled outside his rightful time and place and returned with the memory of jindaleh covering the hillsides in spring, but no one to listen to an Ancient Mariner's story.

"You must come to see Korea today," urged Yoon Bai. "You would be amazed at the changes."

No, I tell him. No use my going to Korea now. It wouldn't be there.

The conversation was conducted in primitive Korean, as much as I was able, then in English. The Japanese speaks only his native language, so my East Asian tongue got saddled up and taken for a bumpy ride.

Yoon Bai's wife is pregnant with twins, he announces proudly. I asked him if there had been a time when such multiple births were thought shameful, litterlike. There was a pause, a shy smile, a dismissive wave of the hand.

"Oh, maybe long, long ago. Not so now."

I did not relate the incident of the murdered twins, which I experienced, and which I have written about in my novel.

Gazing out my bedroom window, I saw—could it be?—the unmistakable wavy flight—*volatu undoso*—of a woodpecker. I had thought it way too soon for them to have returned, but the opening and closing of its wings at every stroke, the rising and falling in curves, is diagnostic. It is a good sign.

Lovely sunny warm day yesterday after the long rain of the day before. Went to the Center for British Art. It was the day after the death of Paul Mellon, who founded the Yale Center for British Art. Saw the Henry Moore sculptures, Lucian Freud's etchings, and the paintings of Francis Bacon, all stunning, powerful. Also a filmed interview of Bacon in which he appears as a charming, candid man who shed a great deal of light on his work. All three of these artists are Ishmaelites, a separate breed with each his different aim. These are men who travel alone in the wilderness of the imagination, friendless, seeing no one; hunters as opposed to tillers of fields and builders of villages. They are especially vulnerable to assassination by the civilized. It is a rare temperament that will strive so mightily in solitude against a cruel and capricious society that wishes them ill. Bacon especially is the natural infidel among the faithful. It is a wonder that, hated as he has been, he did not return that hatred but offered his art as an act of love and generosity.

Feeling not very well still, with productive cough, anorexia, and weakness. Janet too. It is a pest house. I remember a woman years ago at the hospital standing by the stretcher where a young man lay, gasping, pale. She might have been painted by Picasso, her face pulled in opposite directions at once, shattered, the parts dislocated. And not long ago, another Pietà in East Rock Park by the Mill River, where a young woman sat on the grass bending over her guitar, her long hair falling. From the instrument, muted chords that seemed to come from far off. Her lips were parted in song. She was utterly absorbed, as if the struggle to play and sing perfectly were a matter of life and death. Her outline was soft, of no color at all, as if drawn with a loving pencil. I knew, without hearing, that her song was sad, a ballad perhaps. Her eyes streamed, like those of a face made of painted wood. And just this morning, on a balcony, a woman holding something motionless on her lap. A cat, it turned out. The hand that rested there was like the X-ray of a hand, each bone white, fleshless. After a while its tail lifted, swayed.

Shades of Noah's Ark at the Lizzie yesterday. So many crowding into the vault that it began to list whenever the hippos shifted. I was gazed at with the kind of awe habitual to that fierce angel who barred the way back to Eden for Eve. Okay with me, as I prize undeserved renown above all else. S.D. and four other members of the Christian Crusade (Princeton chapter) arrived. I gave them a tour of the Lizzie, served them tea, showed them the vault, then sent them off to evangelize among the heathen. One had read my piece "Abortion" seven years ago and could still recite it chapter and verse! They burned to find out where I stand vis-à-vis Jesus Christ (if I may be immodest). All five are big, good-looking boys who give every outward appearance of normalcy and have no idea that they are bigoted, exclusive, narrow, and fanatic. It is my chance to shake the foundation a tiny bit, if only for a few moments. Their desire to like me and approve of me won out over their suspicions. It won't last more than two blocks.

So much falls away from the sick: ambition, sexual desire, wit, competitive spirit, hobbies, personality. Only left after a while: the primitive secret self of terror, pain, helplessness that was there all the time but covered up with veils of living.

M. in full rave. The missive barrage has resumed with daily letters, tapes, gifts. She has phoned the house twice, the library three times looking for me. Babbling, incoherent. It is a fact that in her madness, she has focused on me, but I cannot be her last resort, her island in a wild sea. On the phone I took the firmest stand. Whatever is to become of this demented woman for whom there is no treatment?

This diary seems a good deal tamer than "The Corpse," "Slaughter-house," and other pieces of time past. I don't at all resent those honest readers who deplore the preoccupation with the morbid that they see as the essential focus of my earlier writing. It is their opinion, and they are entitled to it. And they are welcome to it, for it isn't mine. I am not at all of a morbid cast of mind or taste, only driven to strip away disguises to show the brutal reality of things. Let the squeamish stand back. This is not to say that I don't enjoy shocking people. I do. It's a holdover from boyhood, when I delighted in causing my elders to shake their heads in sorrow and disappointment—wrath, even. With the passage of years, perhaps I have become less curious about the decay and putrefaction that are the destiny of the flesh, and more curious about dream, myth, art.

The weather has turned unusually congenial for this time of year. Still, one remains on guard for a burst of some sort. Best carry an umbrella and keep to oneself. Last evening I attended a lecture by a neurosurgeon on the life of Harvey Cushing, the "father" of neurosurgery. Despite the obligatory worshipfulness, Cushing came across as a *monster sacre* quite of the ilk of my own professors of surgery: ill-tempered, vain, unscrupulous in rivalry, haughty, and godish. One is happy not to have known him, while at the same time one is grateful for his achievements. Thinking about how similar he was to my own chief of surgery, I was reminded of Coventry Patmore's couplet in "The Unknown Eros":

> Yon strives their Leader, lusting to be seen.
> His leprosy's so perfect that men call him clean!

Weeks would go by without a word of praise or an expression of human warmth, lest the chief end by spoiling us brutes. Any slight doubt that he had supreme authority was enough to rouse him to fury. My own situation was particularly onerous. Wit is a scarcity among surgeons—by and large we are as mute as grass—except for myself. I had a modicum of raillery that thrust me into the disgusting role of court jester to that *vil raz di cortigiani*, Rigoletto's vile race of courtiers.

Recuperating from flu, though still with teeth of pearl and breath of lilies. Spent after a haircut, fit only to lie in a canoe on the Mill River (someone else paddling) trailing a finger in the eddy. It being February, I shall sit by the fire recalling the happy time when pipe and pouch were à la mode. It seems that I have always reminisced. In the bassinette I was doubtless recalling the pleasures of the womb, lamenting the clangor and abrasions of life on the outside. As for any writing this week, I have not sown, therefore I shall not reap. Tomorrow will be different, *unberufen*. Having lived since December in the company of contagion, I have learned to carry it lightly. I do not cough in public and conceal the effort not to; I do not shake hands but clap shoulders in greeting; and above all, I go on with the daily routine, lunch with cronies, row at the gym, tea at the Lizzie, just as if I were *valid*.

Professor Minakata dined with us last evening. We discussed the phenomenon that the great notions of physics and mathematics occur in one's teens or early twenties. After that it is mostly tinkering. He told me that while the numbers of his papers have not declined, and in fact have increased, they do not compare in quality to his earliest discoveries. But this is so for writers too, especially poets. Swinburne blazed at the beginning of his career, then faded. One wonders if the same fate would have come to Keats had he lived. Had Chekhov lived to write three plays after *The Cherry Orchard*, it is possible that his gold star might have become tarnished. "What about you?" Minakata-san wanted to know. I said that while I could never recapture the artistry of, say, *Mortal Lessons*, I thought I had found detours that led me to other, less rhapsodic panoramas. To which Minakata-san replied, "Me too." But I think it is less likely for a writer to continue in excellence than it is for a scientist or philosopher. Rhapsody is much less durable than reason.

Received congratulations on the street for the continuing fecundity of my hair—as though a mighty prowess were somehow entailed. Then I overheard a man speaking on the telephone.

"I'll be wearing an ankle-length dark coat with an astrakhan collar and a fresh gardenia boutonniere. You can't miss me."

It is regrettable, but true, that clothing dislikes me. The minute I apply any of it to my person it wrinkles, stains, fades, goes runny. I was meant to live in the Garden of Eden, where, like Adam, I could go about in naked honor clad. Anywhere else, I am all in a heap. Like one of the 120-million-year-old Chinese fossils of feathered dinosaurs at the Peabody Museum, I am bones, beak, and feathers in need of arrangement.

The graduate students are aging before my eyes as their years of peonage go on and on. The hirsute have gone bald, the erect have gone stooped, the slender are sacculate. Gone all freshness and dew. In its place, a cynical wit. I asked a Russian graduate student how long he'd been at it. "This is my seventh year," he said in Boris Godunov bass. "It is not to my advantage to finish too early." Will he be deported should he cease to be a student?

❧

A triumph at the Medical School, where some hundred students packed the Beaumont Room. I told them to gaze and gaze at the human body until what gazes back might be called a soul. Then I read and chattered to warm affection and loud applause, but no one was thoughtful enough to scratch my tummy. My new friend A.C. came along. He reported that my eyes shone with vanity. Together we visited the small study of Harvey Cushing and looked at a fat little volume of his journal full of drawings of the central nervous system, hill towns in Italy, postcards, menus of meals eaten abroad, and all sorts of jottery.

Next morning, after working from 8:30 to 11, I met A.C. at the High Street entrance to the library. We went to the Beinecke to see, and translate, the Gutenberg Bible, thence to the Yale Art Gallery, where he instructed me in nineteenth- and twentieth-century art, about which he is an expert. We shared our lack of enthusiasm for Gauguin. I showed him Eakins's portrait of the veteran, by which he was strangely repulsed.

A.C. is a former recital pianist who now teaches part-time and hates the instrument, preferring to sing in a church choir. His father was an architect and restorer of old churches. He says that he is looking for a wife, but I don't know about that. As a translator he works nonstop from 6 A.M. to 2 A.M. with two fifteen-minute breaks for lunch and supper. He translates three books at a time, as he has three publishers. He rewrites each page many times. "The translator spends more time on a page that the writer," he said.

Well, maybe. In the vault at the Elizabethan Club he admitted to total ignorance of Shakespeare, whom he has never read! I told him that I envied him for what's in store for him. At a quarter to three, exhausted, "Son io spento," I told him. Before parting we lapsed into a vile and salacious exchange. Nothing cements friendship between two men like a descent into the "dirty." After he returned to his own country, I realized that he had made off with my scarf and my cap while he was here in the house, and that it wasn't an accident. A fetishist? One cannot know another person: part of his agenda will always remain out of reach.

Felt bad all day for having declined an invitation by medical students in Kansas City, where I have gone three times in the past eight years. The honorarium consisted of my expenses—as if there were any circumstances under which a speaker would pay his own way. I quickly wrote to decline but I was followed by a day of guilt. Then an anonymous donor offered to pay me a decent wage. Would I change my mind and come? Yes, of course I would. Damn it!

Last night I dreamt that I had gone, as usual, to the Sterling—only it wasn't there. I raced round and round, frantic to find that block of High Street, but it was not to be found, nor did anybody know what happened or why I was upset. It seemed that I was the only one to whom it mattered or for whom it wasn't there. I decided to go somewhere else, but there was nowhere else to go. I felt boneless—*boned*, like a fillet of flounder— and couldn't take a step because my feet had no metatarsals or phalanges.

In the village of Fossacesia, in that part of Italy known as Abruzzi, is the church of San Giovanni e Venere, an odd couple worthy of Ovid. John the Baptist and Venus keeping house (of worship) together? Imagine the ascetic saint and the voluptuous goddess doomed by a mischievous Fate to spend centuries in each other's company. Imagine the old celibate barricading himself in an apse, lest she come, reeking like a civet cat in heat. I have no doubt that sooner or later Venus will have her way with him. The church is a great brooding, hooded pile with a buffalo hump. It sits on the edge of a precipice overlooking the Adriatic Sea. The wall facing east is windowless save for narrow-lidded slits suitable for a fortress—and fortress it had been for much of its later life. The first edifice was of gleaming marble with columns, portico, statuary—your usual Roman version of a Greek temple. With the Christianizing of Rome and the obligatory intolerance of one faith for any other, the Temple of Venus was pulled down and the Romanesque church put up in its place. Today it is undisturbed, save for the goats of the Abruzzesi that browse in the cloister. A few Passionist brothers with a taste for rock and roll live on the premises. In the cloister, portions of the ancient marble columns are still present, and a marble sarcophagus, too. Venus is still very much there. Her smell! In the crypt of San Giovanni e Venere there is a fading fresco showing Jesus and four of the Apostles, one of whom is the very John the Baptist who lives out of wedlock with the Goddess of Love.

Annie Dillard sent her new book. An intriguing marriage of statistics and philosophy. Wrote to thank her.

Lunch at Educated Burgher. It is less a place to eat than it is a deep, narrow wound in the north face of Broadway. It is owned and run by a Greek family with the addition of a counter helper and (behind a door at the rear) one or two Hispanic washers-up. It is a place devoid of pretension. The sighs of the revolving ceiling fans lend a melancholy note to the business conducted below. The upper walls are lined with bookshelves full of books, way out of arm's reach but giving a touch of conviction to the word *Educated*. Booths for four and tables for two are each supplied with an ashtray. Smoking is not frowned upon except for the very rear, where there is a sign to that effect, which no one seems to read. The hot animal smell of hamburgers and hot dogs is stirred by the fans. No sooner inside the door, when one of the two counter staff will call out "Help someone?" in a tone of voice that lets you know you'd better be ready to order. Out of sheer intimidation, I always get the soup du jour. On Friday there is a clam chowder that could receive compliments in Heaven. When I can gather my wits, I add to that a hot dog or a cup of chili. Other times, I slink out and get a slice of pizza next door, but not without a feeling of guilt. The service is "self," with a centrally located bar for ketchup, mustard, relish, and chopped onions.

The food is tasty and cheap, the menu unalterable but sufficiently diverse. Overall it strikes a note of contempt for the cholesterol level and atherosclerosis of its clientele. The clientele is eclectic and includes construction workers, postmen, moviegoers, Yalies, the elderly fixed-income crowd, and an assortment of the odd outscourings of the human race. These, the lumpish, the gnarled, the dwarfed, the morbidly obese, the mentally disheveled, are all treated with the same phlegm as the occasional alumnus who drops in unawares. As would be the mayor or the president of Yale. At the Educated Burgher, if nowhere else, rank hath no privileges; it is classic hash-house democracy in action. Not long ago, I shared a table with a woman eating a hamburger deluxe. With every mouthful, she rolled her eyes up into her skull. I tried manfully not to notice. There is almost always a former patient of mine who simply cannot refrain from announcing to all within earshot that I had made a "deep impression" on him, then splitting his sides. I can say, without the least hesitation, that Educated Burgher is my favorite luncheonette, although I would not dare to use that word on the premises.

Attended a panel discussion on "the museum" by the director of the Yale Art Gallery's British Art Collection, an art historian and a disciple of Josef Albers, in whose memory the conclave was being held. Did I know him? Only in the peripheral sense. I recall excising a malignant tumor from his foot and doing a skin graft, all the while he studied in silence the place where the yellow wall met the white ceiling.

In the matter of museums, the earliest were caves whose walls were used by the artists. Elevations and declivities of the stone were made use of to define a haunch. The paintings were seen only by firelight, which must have given the illusion of motion to the animals. How perfect this was for the people of that time! Their achievement seems to me no less than all that has come in the millennia of museums since. I should far rather be lowered into a cave at Lascaux than stand in line at the Uffizi. Further evidence that, unlike science, there is no such thing as progress in art.

⁊☙

Reflected upon the fact that there is a kind of genius in merely turning seventy. Then hailed the Muse. "Erato, come!" But she remained as silent as the stare of a barn owl. By midafternoon, my head had filled with helium. Went to the gym.

At age twelve, I looked in the mirror and saw a strange, sad, ecstatic face with eyes that were gray-green marbles flecked with gold. The pale skin turned violet beneath those eyes. The chin, mouth, and nose had the look of a small animal's snout, one of those nervous creatures of the under-brush, always crouching—a chipmunk.

If there is one thing I have done that is right and perfect, it is my son Jon. Those dear children! They all go off to the south of France for a week to play in the sand, precisely what I would like to do instead of mounting a half-dozen podia in Sacramento.

My turn to do the marketing. I came home from Ferraro's with a length of turkey sausage, a pineapple, a frozen octopus, six large beets, and four artichokes. Janet unwrapped the packages.

"I see," she remarked thoughtfully, "let's put it all in a big pot, boil it up and call it 'The Last Supper.'"

"*Ingrata!*" I muttered. Besides, I do too know what to do with that octopus. First, you put it in a big pot and boil it. (She got that part right.) After an hour, you skin the thing, then you have a choice: either cut it up for salads, add it to tomato sauce, or marinate and grill. I'm leaning toward the last. Don't worry, she'll come salivating, all right. One must not wince, but brace oneself for the slings and arrows of the insensitive.

Snow. Lots of it during the night. Saint Ronan Terrace has a certain mortuary charm. The city itself is a necropolis where no one stirs and everything lies buried. Every branch and twig laden. The birds arranged themselves as calligraphy. I tried reading the message but before I could, they had turned the page and flew off, twittering. Walked to Mill River. Two swans taking off. What a beating they gave to the startled air!

Began the octopedal enterprise. Simmered the creature in water, garlic, bay leaf, salt, and pepper for more than an hour. Stuck it with a knife. It went in easily. Made a marinade with teriyaki sauce, wine, and fish sauce. There it shall welter overnight. Tomorrow, to the grill!

About the octopus, I refuse to be modest. A sublimity. Even the creature would have been delighted to offer himself for such a feast.

My notebook smells of garlic.

The snow has melted, every bit. And there they were—last year's yellow pansies in full bloom. But then they have bloomed all winter long. The vanity of it! Or the stupidity of these flowers.

You can't guess what went hopping by me on Hillhouse Avenue this morning. A frog! Green as the eyes of a vampire. In March! Whence came it? And whither hoppeth? But there it was, and no one to share it with. Only a squirrel, who sat up, cocked his head, and covered his eyes with his paws. He couldn't believe it either.

Decided to give William Carlos Williams one more chance out of simple Christian charity. Reread half a dozen of his doctor stories, and no, I can live very well without W.C.W. They are slapdash and carelessly wrought. I would rattle his pedestal.

Bought a slice (to go) at Broadway Pizza, took it to the island of pavement and brick that lies between Broadway and Elm. There are stone benches there, just right for dining al fresco. All of a sudden, a cry: "Hey, Dad!" Gretchen driving by. What a sight for a daughter—in my scuffed shoes, tattered black vest, baggy corduroys, and wild thatch of gray. Just me and my elderly briefcase having a picnic between two lines of traffic. You can't imagine the purgative pleasure of such a slice, even with a side dish of exhaust fumes. I forgot to mention the three pigeons who waited at table from a respectful distance.

Sat right down and began to write the introduction to the nonfiction book. It opens in Troy, naturally, and pleasurable it is to sift the ashes of memory. No chewing of the pen in anguish, no gashing the paper. I'll pay for it, surely. One has to pay for even this small happiness. Soon enough, an interruption by one of the loonies. They are slowly making the library uninhabitable. I must pray for more tolerance.

⁂

Yesterday I was put in charge of Beck and Lulu (Lucy) for the afternoon while Janet prepared for the dinner party (our one per year). We went for ice cream, then to East Rock Park, where we sailed stickboats on the Mill River, stood under the waterfall to feel the spray on our faces, skipped flat stones, wrote our names on trees, in sand, in water, and ignored the gloom of the trees. So many elderly corpses lying about. Home, with them in a state of high excitement, and I in one of exhaustion.

⁂

The mourning doves, cardinals, blue jays and woodpeckers are all over the yard. Everything with wings is in full throat.

⁂

Awake and hungry at three in the morning. Read a novel by Natalia Ginzburg, an amusing Italian writer. Lay there thinking about breakfast. Should I have my egg scrambled or hard boiled? That sort of thing. Got up and boiled an egg, remembering that I'm not allowed to eat the yoke. Continued reading the novel until time to bring in the newspapers at five o'clock. Read about the Kosovo debacle, the ethnic cleansing there, and the prospect of war.

⁂

Tapping away at the *Troy* sequel. Perhaps it is worthy, perhaps not. In the twenties and thirties in that fabled town one still lived on the cusp of what was called "progress." There was, of course, electricity, but the smell of candlewax was everywhere. Automobiles, yes—grog-eyed, dashed, and fendered—but in the streets horse manure gilded the cobblestones. Coal still had to be shoveled, the furnace stoked, the mysteries of the damper solved. The Industrial Revolution had long since been born, but we were its long-delayed afterbirth.

I have been gazing at Mark Rothko's *No. 3* at the Yale Art Gallery and looking into his work for one of my art lectures. Thus far it seems to me that the paintings of Rothko are claustrophobic, closed off, blocked from the viewer, impoverished. They refer back only to themselves and are alienated from everything that is human. As for the rendering of the spiritual, give me a human face.

Strange things are happening. I was sitting in the courtyard at the Sterling, eating a sandwich, when I heard a frantic squeak overhead and looked up to see a hawk with a not-yet-dead squirrel in its talons. The hawk made it to the edge of the roof, where I could see it feasting. The squirrel's tail hung over the edge and flapped in the wind so as to make you think it was still alive. In a moment, a squadron of crows began dive-bombing the hawk, but it fed on, unconcerned. Minutes later a helicopter came near, too near for the hawk, who abandoned his meal and soared off with the crows mobbing after him.

Then this. For over a week, lying on the table in the Computer Room at the Sterling, there has been a book, *Introduction to the Yoruba Language*, along with a student's notebook. Each day I have waited for the student to appear and reclaim it. For the past few days I have been . . . well . . . *studying* it, doing the assignments. I can say things like "I am hot," "Rain is coming down on me," "The harmattan is here now," "I am suffering from the harmattan." The harmattan is the West African trade wind that carries a lot of dust, makes man and beast irritable, and combines with monsoons to cause tornadoes. Some susceptible people fall ill with fever during the harmattan. What can it all mean? Am I going to take a trip to Nigeria for birdwatching? If so, I shall make sure it is not the time of the harmattan; I am positive that I would be susceptible.

Other news: a Dutch translator whom I met while he was visiting Yale for a book about Boswell has read my books and writes that he wants to translate *all* of them into Dutch. Last year Spain and Chile; this year Japan; next year the Netherlands. Little by little, country by country, I am taking over the world. Already I have had two attacks of megalomania.

I am putting my talk on the Yale Pietà into the computer. I haven't yet had the nerve to inform the Yale Art Gallery that their works are to be reproduced in a book. They'll probably rise up in high dudgeon, and I'll be led away in manacles, made to sit on the stool of Repentance.

It is moving to watch a hen crouch over her chicks, flap her bony wings, and squawk when a hawk circles above. It is even more moving to watch her do this when what soars overhead is not a raptor but a kite made of paper and sticks. The one is in the natural scheme of predation and survival. It must be accepted. But in the second, there is added the element of black comedy to a mother's frenzy. This is far more compelling to a writer.

Spring is rampant hereabouts, in full upthrust. Those insane pansies that have never stopped blooming all through the winter have washed their faces and are greeting the dwarf tulips, snowdrops, hyacinths, and daffodils. All around the house this morning I hear woodpeckers, mourning doves, cardinals. At dusk, owls. The fur of the raccoon is spotless. A crow bore a large twig overhead. A full moon quivered in the sky like a reflection in a pool of water. Spring, and I am missing tobacco again.

This afternoon I met a charming Korean OB/GYN, here at Yale for two years as a post doc. A new bus-stop friend. Spoke the language so as to dazzle him and stupefy myself. One of those rare moments when phrases came flooding back. "I am Christian," he announced, and told me how every morning, before going to work, he goes to church to pray to God. As he said this, he put his palms together and bowed his head. When he raised it, his perfect white teeth gleamed. It is Good Friday, and heaven was looking over our shoulders, because the shuttle bus didn't come, and we had to walk together for fifteen minutes. His name, of course, is Jang—the name of Dr. Sloane's loyal assistant in my Korean novel.

I no longer think of disease in terms of statistics. I think only of its uniqueness. The doctor is eyewitness to someone else's nightmare.

Why I use language of a "high" style rather than quotidian. It is honorific. In telling the story of a patient, it is my duty to sing of his suffering in words worthy of its greatness. The way Homer sang of Achilles or Odysseus. In the Korean language, there are four ways to say everything to another person. The highest is the formal, or honorific, and is used toward someone who is old or respected.

The human body may need the help of a doctor to realize its potential.

In less than 48 hours I leave for Sacramento. From the fuss I'm making about it, you'd think I was heading for Babylonia. I don't mind saying that I don't want to go, and I'm scared to death about all those talks I have to give. I have a vision of my mouth in constant rubbery motion, with all sorts of rejectimenta spilling onto my chin and vest. Yesterday I went to a talk about an eighteenth-century female letter writer, Madame de Graffigny. The talk was given by an attractive young feminist who spoke on orgasm in the elderly female and on bowel and bladder function in the same. I was greatly amused at the discomfiture of the dignified male French professors in the audience. I am now reading Madame de Graffigny's letters—she wrote 2,500 of them to a gay friend many years her junior. They're in French, as was the lecture, so I probably miss a lot.

I still have the taste and temperament of a surgeon and the gaze of diagnosis and prediction. Every evening I take the Yale shuttle bus home. I think now of that elderly Chinese man I saw sitting on the opposite side of the bus one row in front of me. He looked a tiny figurine, really, made of old yellow ivory and wax. He was so thin that I could see the calcified artery that throbbed in his left temple, and so precisely did this blood vessel present itself under the papery skin that I could count the rhythm of its pulsation and diagnosed auricular fibrillation. This is an irregular beat that is fatal in 20 percent of cases. Suddenly, an ethical dilemma. Should I reach across, tap the man on the shoulder, and say, "Excuse me, Sir, but you have a heart condition, and you need to see a doctor"? Perhaps he didn't speak English. Perhaps he was under a doctor's care already. Perhaps he would think me meddlesome and rude. Just then the bus pulled up to my stop and I got off. Ever since, I have regretted my inaction.

How difficult it has become for us to define the human body, what with the transplantation of organs from one individual to another and even one species to another. Add to this the practice of plastic and cosmetic surgery, sex-change operations, the implantation of genes from mice and pigs to man, in vitro fertilization, gene therapy, and there is plenty of room for skepticism about the sacredness of the human body, which has been violated at every turn. Something within me recoils from the technological reductio ad absurdum of the body. As I have often said, some mysteries are not meant to be solved, they are meant to be deepened. While I have never believed in the Resurrection of the Flesh—that we shall be raised for the Last Judgment intact, *ipso corpore* (this very flesh)— I am drawn to the notion of the human body as unique and infinitely variable. If that is what is meant by sacred, then yes, I do hold to the holiness of the flesh.

Today I went to Saint Mary's Church for Easter Sunday Mass. Stood at the rear of the filled church so as not to occupy a seat better taken by a real Catholic. On either side of the central aisle, candles inside gleaming hurricane lamps adorned every other pew. The alternates wore bouquets of fresh flowers. Splendid music, especially a dark mezzo-soprano who sang mostly solo. The procession passed by me, and Carleton Jones, pastor, smiled at me in mild surprise. I recognized one of the acolytes as a graduate student. I was bowled over by the pageantry. Incense. Readings from Saint Paul and Saint Matthew. Carleton's sermon was on the subject of fear. The fear inspired in his disciples by Christ from which only he could release them. The fear that is the instrument of the devil and that keeps us all from believing in Christ, and from leading a good life—for example, having an abortion or committing euthanasia out of fear. I left before Communion as there is a limit to my tolerance and my imposturage. Stepped outside into the light of New Haven with my skepticism reinforced.

I read in the *New York Times* that I am an old-fashioned writer. What with my fountain pen and notebook, I do feel quite quaint, as though I had lived in 1899, with gas lamps in the streets, oil lamps indoors, a horsehair mattress on the bed, and a chamber pot beneath it. I am sure I give off a faint odor comprised of tobacco, old leather, and dead roses. Other days I feel quite lusty and make outrageous remarks to women. Why only this morning I was greeted by a woman I don't know, and I asked her name in return. "Never mind," she said. "Everyone knows you, Doctor Selzer. You don't have to know us." At which I felt a surge of childish vanity. I went to the gym, where the men were not noticeably virile, being porky and soft-looking—although that's hardly a reliable measure. Still, I palpated with a blend of pride and disdain over my flat stomach and bony elbows. Another surge of vanity.

On the flight from O'Hare to Sacramento, which was delayed for two hours, I sat next to a charming light-skinned African American boy of eight. First he offered me a stick of gum. After listening to the stewardess give instructions for an emergency landing, he said, "Don't worry. God is watching over us." When I went to eat my lunch, he stopped me until I clasped my hands and joined him in saying grace. In return, I showed him how to make the veins in his hands stand out, then disappear, and I taught him how to feel his own radial pulse. Whereupon he announced his decision to become a doctor. He has never seen his father, doesn't know where he is. He and his brother were adopted by a white woman in the row behind us. "You are my friend," he said. "No, *you are my grandfather*." At which the elastic ball of my heart bounced at his feet.

Last night I gave the final talk. The affair was held in a grotesque Chinese restaurant called the Fat House. (Fat is the owner's name.) I had planned to present "Yale's Ivory Christ" as an example of physical diagnosis, for which I had brought slides of the sculpture—but when I saw that room! There was an artificial waterslide at my back, audible music—all the clackery and chop suey of China—so I changed plans at the last instant and read "A Worm from My Notebook," which was severely under-rehearsed. Anyway, the podiocy ordeal is over, and I am the darling of the Davis Medical establishment. Doubtless everybody, of all genders and species, desired to get into bed with me, but I stupidly never gave one iota of encouragement, so I have been me and me-ing it.

This morning I moved a vase of lilies into the kitchen, placed it on a waist-high shelf, then sat under the lily tree to sip my morning coffee. Any wanton who dares to do this is in danger of losing all composure and being swept away on a wave of lubricity, for to some the scent of the lily is sharp, edgy, *sexual*. Madame Bovary, for one. She fell into a state of "mystic lassitude" (read *erotomania*) from the perfume exhaled by lilies at a religious fête. In fact the lily was the symbolic flower of Aphrodite and was adopted for the Virgin Mary. No depiction of the Annunciation is complete without a vase of lilies on the shelf, or hovering in midair. And the several million Susannahs, Susans, and Shoshanas of the world might not know that their name is the Hebrew word for purity and synonymous with the word for lily. But why does the lily droop its blossoms, bowing its head? Surely not out of modesty. In shame, rather. Pope said that it's for Saint Catherine that they hang their heavy heads and die. Of course death is symbolized by the pallor of the lily, just as love is symbolized by the ardor of the rose. But in Rubrum lily the two coexist in their most violent embrace. The bound feet of the Chinese women were referred to as golden waterlilies. Lily-footed means *bound*.

Aside from Noah, the only sympathetic character in the Old Testament is Isaiah, who interspersed his conversations with Jehovah with complaints about his bowels, comparing his cramps to labor pains:

My loins are filled with anguish,
Pangs have seized me
Like the pangs of a woman in travail.
I am bowed down so that I cannot hear,
I am dismayed so that I cannot see.

And again Isaiah exclaims:

My bowels resound like a harp.

May-ah-yim is Hebrew for bowels; *Kah-kee-nohr* is the word for harp.
Such a careful reading convinces me that the old prophet was suffering
from spastic colitis. "Listen to the patient," taught Sir William Osler. "He
is trying to tell you what is the matter with him."

I haven't found any of *my* friends in the Old Testament.

In a diary you can quote or misquote the Bible, Proust, Dante. You can
drop in as much Latin, Greek, French, or Japanese as makes you feel
good. And a diary is the repository for your secret heresies. Here are four
of mine:

1) William Carlos Williams had little, if any, talent—two or three rather
good poems, the rest a gigantic literary scam. Mostly he is a poet by typo-
graphical courtesy alone—the arrangement of the words on the page. Besides, he was not a nice man. But I've said all this before. Got hell for it, too.

2) *Moby-Dick* would have been a much better novel had Melville cut
it to 250 pages.

3) Much as I love nature, I can't read Wordsworth—he makes me
sick.

4) As for Walt Whitman, take out all the bombast, the lists, the
ecstatic flying spittle, the lyric apostrophes, and what's left *could* be poetry—I'm not sure.

First morning of birdwatching in East Rock Park. All the old friends there. I adore those who watch birds as much as I adore that which they watch. And my skull was full of palm warblers, ruby-crowned kinglets, black and whites, yellow rumps—all the way from ophryon to inion.

Off to Providence in a few hours. The podiocist is not unlike the exile or the refugee. The way he drifts back and forth across North America spending nights and days in hotels, B&Bs, and hospices, where he is called, with cruel irony, a guest. The podiocist is forever en route. The destination hardly matters, only the point of departure, for the object is to escape from what is perceived as a repression, a yoke. And so every morning, one must lug one's mulish valise aboard yet another vehicle and be hurtled to yet another station. It should come as no surprise that the podiocist's grasp on reality is shaky. What day of the week is it? He doesn't know. What month? He shrugs. What is the currency of this place—lire, shekels? As for the cuisine, well . . . Never mind; punch-drunk from decades of podiocy, he'll eat anything. A lot depends on the weather. If it is raining, he travels into the past. Should the sun be shining along his route, there are apt to be premonitions, déja vus, trances, daydreams, and those privileged moments that offer a glimpse of the future.

Of course, I know that I don't have to go, that I can refuse these invitations to speak. You don't have to tell me that. But how else would you have me earn a living? *Ich kann nicht anders,* in the words of Martin Luther. Besides, how do you know what pain or sorrow I dart and zigzag to dodge? No, it's the podiocist's curse that he is free to release himself from the "Road" at any time, but will not. It is a self-imposed punishment overlooked by Dante.

Of course, I know too that I shouldn't record each one of my ovations, not even in this notebook. But I'm as vain as the next. And as pathetic.

Met with students. (They follow me around the library, stand apart until I motion them to come on over.) Had once told them that writing is not living but one step removed from life. Why write, then, asked a lickable girl (an inspired typo). Clarified that while writing is not the same as living, it is not a rung lower than life but higher at certain moments of creativity. Call it rapture. Also, it thrills me to think that through the permanence of art, I may come into the presence of generations of people to come. If that is an unrealistic expectation, why so be it. The very possibility sustains me. Asked by another, rather less appetizing, about the rivalry, competitiveness, and jealousy among writers. Said, Nothing could be more stupid or self-destructive. A waste of time. If a work is worthy of being preserved, it will be kept. If not, it will be forgotten. No amount of elbowing or nudging will have the least effect. (Class dismissed with a wave of a pencil.)

Jon Schueler's lifelong search, both in life and art, is for a woman. Or Woman. But she is just out of his reach. It is the striving to grasp her that is the prima stamina (he claims) of his painting. Rage, loneliness, and sexual deprivation provide the energy for his art. To me, this is a foreign language in which I am iliterate. The only woman who has been a presence in my writing is the woman inside myself, that part of me which is a woman. This is said with no embarrassment, and in all honesty. Schueler's quest is in the line of Dante, Petrarch, Yeats—a noble tradition. By page 118, however, I begin to mistrust Jon Schueler. Altogether too much whining, breast-beating, self-regarding. For all his great success with women, there is an unmanliness about him.

Janet and I walked to the summit of East Rock Park. Dogwood in bloom all the way. Lovely clear day. On such a morning matrimony does not seem so arduous an affair.

The weather—rain, fog—has done in the birdwatching. Doon and I are desolate but bearing up. Swell tête-à-tête with him in the park. He is a marvelous human being. Took him to lunch with the Boys Friendly, where he was idolized by the emeriti. Pop thrilled.

I have gone birdwatching all week for four hours every morning with my son Doon. I am horribly fit, having clambered up and down the mountain of East Rock, leaping from crag to crag. But today the family has left, and I have one day to prepare to go to Kansas City, where I'm to give two talks, and try to console my friend K. for having lost his surgical priv-ileges at the hospital, and probably all over. That's the way it works. I don't know the real reason for it, but he is quite demolished.

"This about you?"

It was a young faculty member in the Medical School famous for his smirk. He held up a copy of *What One Man Said to Another*.

"A tissue of lies," I told him, "made up just to be congenial."

"Sure it is," said the professor in the poisonous voice of a youth who disapproves of one simply because one has grown old. "All my friends are waiting to read it too."

"Ayez pitié de moi!" I implored as the lout sauntered off with my honor in his hip pocket.

Returned to my carrel, closed the door, and turned out the light, informing patient and pilgrim alike that "The Doctor Is Out." Sat there for half an hour, my skull as "dry as the remainder biscuit after a voyage."

During lunch with the Boys Friendly, much hilarity over a line in John Marston's play *The Malcontent*. One character refers to an Irishman's hatred of bumcracks. George Hunter, who edited this Elizabethan drama, explained that if you farted in the presence of an Irishman, he would draw his dagger and kill you.

Here's how it goes. After a night of broken sleep (I awaken every two hours—the prostatic curse), I rise from the bed at five and prepare breakfast: white of a hardboiled egg + slice of bread + butter + a bit of cream cheese + 3 cups of black coffee (no sugar). Also grapefruit juice to wash down three pills (one tiny pink one, one aspirin, and one rough coffin-shaped gray). I do this not out of any conviction that it does me good but to placate the gods of Supplementary Ingestion. Then I retrieve the newspapers from the foot of the driveway and skim the *New York Times* and the *New Haven Register,* both of which I would shred had I the power. At 6:45 Janet comes down and I go upstairs to write a few letters, shower, and leave for the library, before which there is a strategy session at which we both plan the day. I generally walk the twenty minutes to the library down Hillhouse Avenue. Am I early? Then I stop at the Yale Computer Cluster on that street and deal with e-mail. If not, I go directly to the Sterling and begin. My task now is to prepare the nonfiction book for which a contract is being written (a measly contract, but nothing to do about that). I have three of the art lectures ready for typing. The fourth, *"The Dying Centaur,"* is for tomorrow and the day after. Meanwhile, this weekend is Commencement, and New Haven is bursting!

Commencement Day at Yale. I much prefer its opposite: Termination. Just the sight of all the Moms and Pops bursting with pride and trying to conceal their exhaustion gives one cause to wax either sentimental or cynical—or in my case, both. This morning I'm to meet with a former student at the Medical School with whom I had been very close for the year that he was assigned to me. He's arguably the handsomest Yalie of all time, captain of the football team, brilliant, dexterous—all of that, and he was aiming for a career in surgery. Boom! He fell under the spell of the Jehovah's Witnesses and converted to that faith. The local leader and I competed for the student, even going so far as to engage in debates, both public and private. The student dropped out to devote himself to missionary work. I was quite cast down over it. He went on to become a very successful building contractor, spending most of his time and money among the Witnesses, building their Meeting Halls and such. Every few years he comes to see me—I can't think why. He has always needed to keep me in his pocket, for he worries that I will dismiss him. In fact I have. But there is about him something that I don't know, an inner disturbance to which I have unknowingly contributed. Perhaps I'm a stand-in for his rigid, blue-collar father, who is a Roman Catholic? Has he been a bit in love with me? Does he have regrets about leaving medicine and Catholicism for this "marginal" faith? I'm still guessing twenty years later. He'll never say what it is, although I've given him every chance. This morning I'll try again. All of which confirms my belief that biography is stupid. No one knows anything about anyone else. I have read four biographies of Chekhov, but he remains a mystery, having eluded his biographers entirely. I plan to do the same should the dreadful occasion ever arise.

A good day at the desk, then read two stories by Chekhov and had a slice of pizza al fresco alongside but not *with* construction workers and pigeons. I shrink to intrude upon the conviviality of the one and the insatiable hunger of the other.

The way something is said may be the determining difference between the facts and what some might question as the truth. A neurologist might speak of epilepsy as the discharge of erratic impulses in the brain, often related to a lesion such as a scar or a tumor. A writer might try to render the condition from the epileptic's point of view: he had the feeling that something in his head had come loose and was yawing wildly from side to side—a wobble of the temporal lobe. Does the use of metaphoric language make the writer's rendition any less true? I think it does not, and in this instance it offers the nonepileptic reader a sensation to which he can relate.

If only there were a God to thank for this lovely life of literary seclusion. Today I sat in the garden at dawn and wrote two letters in each of which I strewed a pinch of airs and graces. This afternoon I walked through a grove of linden trees in Farnum gardens behind the house. O the scent! I think of a line by the Scottish poet William Aytoun: "When the bees have ceased to murmur in the umbrage of the lime" (in the U.K., the linden tree is called the lime).

Sunday I attended the unveiling for Janet's Aunt Sadie, at which the rabbi read from a work of the Apocrypha. It had to do with the error of allowing grief or pain to dominate one's life. Later the rabbi showed me a sentence he had omitted: "Death is preferable to continued suffering or grief." Left it out, he explained, as it was upsetting to some to be told at the gravesite not to go on grieving. Also, he'd seen *A Question of Mercy* and knew where I stood on assisted suicide.

Awoke and wished myself Happy Birthday, then let my seventy-one-year-old mind caracole where it would. I decided to begin assembling the Rothko piece for the Yale Art Gallery. The day's work having been decided, I made coffee, boiled an egg, ate cold pineapple, and set off to the Sterling with not a care in the world. I was stopped by a Yale cop and a Yale gardener in succession, each needing to tell me about his mental pain. I broke free and on down Prospect. As I crossed Beinecke Plaza I thought of how the other day a sudden downpour had driven me inside the Rare Books and Manuscripts Library. The marbles of the building had turned rain-colored, but minutes later the sun returned and then the marbles flamed. The Beinecke is an animal gifted with camouflage that takes on the hue and pattern of its environs in order to escape notice. At the Sterling I held office hours. Harry, a security guard, announced that his urine was very dark. I checked his sclera and saw no sign of icterus. Anything else? Yes, he's been having nightsweats, so I sent him for urinalysis, CBC, and liver function tests. I spent three hours on Rothko, then to lunch on pea soup and pizza, thinking about a phone call from Troy, one of two partners who lived at 45 Second Street some years ago and had invited me to visit my natal home again. Now they have started a small theater group called Nickel and Dime and in October will do a reading of *A Question of Mercy*. Would I come to comment and help raise money? It's as good an excuse to return to Troy as any. Tomorrow I go there for a nostalgic wallow with my brother Bill.

I admit it: I have a lamentable weakness for the odd outscourings of the human race—the mad, the deformed, and the hugely obese. I squinny at them every chance I get. It is ignoble and not normal, but then I never said that I was. The other day I attended one of those ghastly brunches where you are urged to eat all that you can. In the party was a young woman of several hundred pounds. Well, 250 anyway. I watched as she did away with plate after heaping plateful of food—meat, fish, waffles, salads, pasta, et cetera. To my shame, I followed her to the dessert table, where she filled two large platters with every kind of tart, éclair, cake, pie, and cookie. In full sail and fully laden she was magnificent on the voyage to her seat.

A thousand years ago I wouldn't have needed a pet fool, I would have found myself adequate to the task.

Two days in Troy with brother Bill. Sat on a bench by the river drinking bourbon from plastic cups, watching the Hudson go shouldering by. No one could accuse it of being impetuous or expansive, the way it turns narrow and straight at Troy without the least bit of hilarity.

First came the annual reproach from Bill about my having drifted from all religion and my healthy skepticism about the existence of God. It is the unseemliness of such a stance that bothers him—*it is bad manners*. No use my pointing out that so many are persecuted in this life for having a particular religion and damned in the next for having had none. Next, with the presbyopia of the nostalgic mind, we squinted into focus the distant town of our childhood and its inhabitants all the way back *ab incarnato*. Bill has become a rather paunchy fellow, with opinions up and down. Do the deep sighs that seem to decompress his big belly suggest self-awareness? No, his life is a succession of rich meals, cruises, the stock market, and his sweetheart Rosalie. I am his only friend. The visit is an occasion to disburden himself of a thousand dredged resentments—his face will go fat with them—and moments of remembered glory.

Following Bill up the steps to Tom's house, I watched the working of his shoulderblades. They seemed too small for the massive back they strove to lift. We were in shorts, and I watched his too popliteal vulnerability, the melancholy thing that is his nape with its ancient sebaceous cyst. And then there is Tom, with whom we were staying, a decision I regretted, perhaps because I am simply getting tired. I must pull him up out of a chair, tuck his feet into the car, and untuck them when he alights. Poor Tom, wearing the masklike *facies* of Parkinson's, with shuffling gait and profound weakness. His nose runs all the time—he says it's embarrassing—and he hears nothing that is not shouted down into his ear trumpet (hearing aids don't work). But I *must* stop this infernal dwelling on decrepitude. Tom's all right. His garden would put an Eden to shame. And Bill is rendered goofy at the mention of Rosalie. Also, I am no better off than either of them.

Just returned from two days of sentimental wallow with brother Bill. Difficult, this time. There is no single way in which we are alike. None. Whereas before I could call upon a reserve of familial devotion, I am grown querulous and crotchety. I am distanced by his gluttony, which in the past I had let go as a healthy appetite. I am offended by his bullheaded insistence on being right all the time, where before I accepted it as an antidote to my indecisiveness. His defiant vulgarity (he says *ain't* in every sentence) had once been a harmless mannerism. It is now a measure of his rejection of literature, art, refinement of any kind. His self-absorption is absolute, and he requires my approval of every miscalculation. I give it far more than I withhold it because his need is greater than mine. I think he will die in the arms of Rosalie, so that I needn't feel dread or pain. Nor shall I mourn should he go first. It will just have been *that*.

Lunch with the Boys Friendly evolved into a lighthearted exchange about our infirmities. Louie Martz, poor man, has a herniated nucleus pulposus with sciatic nerve compression. It came after lifting some heavy flowerpots. Louie is eighty-five and married to a woman who is forty-five years younger than he. When she admonished him to act his age, he replied that if he had done that he wouldn't have married her. Then there is the plague of deafness which has the unexpected benefit of causing us to sit close together the way the disciples leaned toward Jesus at the Last Supper (the diarist is Judas). And the other plagues of forgetfulness, cataracts ripe and green, a bit of coronary artery atherosclerosis here and there, and so on. When my turn came I said that I wanted an ailment that would settle down with me like an old family servant, so that we might get to know each other's little ways and make allowances. Something internal, I thought, with which to occupy my mind.

"Like what?"

"Like lactose intolerance. Or spastic colon. Nothing incapacitating, mind you, just the occasional *pffft* of testimony from the bowel. Or maybe RLS."

"Robert Louis Stevenson?"

"No. Restless Leg Syndrome."

We were six old men not in the least embarrassed by the richness of our bodily eccentricities, and, it appeared, moated about by them, as no one stopped at the table to visit.

Thinking about brother Bill, the way he must always be considered successful. His head, though often bloodied, must remain unbowed. Nothing wrong with any of that, I suppose. Then too there is his gluttony. He has the stomach of an ostrich. It can accept anything but rubber tires. Virility is a cheese omelet followed by strawberry pancakes with whipped cream for breakfast. His soul is at least as capacious as his guts. No sooner had I begun the homeward drive than I felt a pang of remorse. Should he fall ill or die, my own irritability and impatience would accuse me forever. He is, after all, a good, kind, soft-hearted man. Besides, all those cherished resentments and animosities are the real ties that bind, aren't they?

As for Rosalie, it is a stupid Talmud that says a man without a woman is not a person, that he is nothing, but certainly Rosalie is the other half of

Bill, and it is no more odd than any other pairing-up of man and woman for life. I listened to an account of a three-week cruise. While Bill gave bridge lessons in return for their passage, Rosalie, beautiful, bejeweled, and bespangled, was the cynosure of all eyes. Aboard ship, three hundred wealthy Jews! Nothing wrong with that, either. Nothing wrong with anything except me. I am all wrong. The visit ended with lunch at a Chinese restaurant. The struggle of a pair of Old Trojans with chopsticks lowers the tone of a meal from tragedy to farce. On the way home I sang "Earth Has No Sorrow That Heaven Cannot Heal," and "Come, Ye Disconsolate," hymns I'd played in Korea for Sunday church services. By the time I got to Waterbury I could no longer see Bill's lumpish face, all bulge and pouch, only the deep cleft in his chin where the angel had touched him.

I looked at a photograph of Bill. It is in his slumberous, fleshy face that both Mother and Father live on. I resemble neither one of them in the least—further evidence, if any were needed, that I am a changeling. But changelings are warm-blooded too. We need love as much as anyone else does. When I was a child I was often told that I was odd, so I became odd, if only to be congenial.

Saint Jon's Day. The family is en route. This will be my last day at the library for the duration of their stay, three weeks. Nor shall I write a line. I don't give a damn if my right hand forgets its cunning. It already has—for the past week the penflux has done nothing but dribble, squirt, and spill, none of which is worth crying over. Spilt ink? Is there anyone still alive who remembers when the ink ran out of the pen of its own volition and you had to use a blotter? *Ink. Blotter.* Are these words still in the language? The other day, at an exhibition of posters from World War I at the Center for British Art, the word *zeppelin* was used repeatedly, causing the young security guard to ask me what it was. I explained in some detail about the gas, hydrogen, that is lighter than air. How it is flammable, and most of the zeppelins exploded and burned—this partly because the Americans wouldn't sell the much safer helium to our allies—can't remember why. From the expression on his face, I might have been describing a medieval catapult or *ballista*.

Only 10:30 in the morning and already I yawn cavernously and commit various acts of pandiculation. Scandalous behavior in a library! But the place is strangely empty. Not a single patient. Not a lump or an earache or even an ingrown toenail. The entire staff and patronage have vanished while I was taking a nap. The loonies too are summering elsewhere.

Spent all day in the library trying to turn myself into a book, only people wouldn't let me—they kept clearing their throats and asking me to feel a lump or look into a mouth or an ear, trim a toenail . . . or simply laying out their sad lives like the entrails of a goat to be examined for signs. No matter how sternly I wave them away or turn my chair, they drift back to me. Perhaps I have chosen my place unwisely. A café might have been more sympathetic than this vast space dotted with the forlorn, the hypochondriacal, and the scholarly. A café, perhaps, with workmen sitting before glasses of grappa or vino, their knobby hands resting on their knobby knees. Let it be a small square where one might feed the squirrels and pigeons with a crust of pizza.

Another tearful farewell after three weeks of Jon, Regine, et al. Danny and Emmy are superb children. This morning I had taken them on an excursion through the Bamboo Forest, planted twenty years ago by their father as a few isolated canes, now grown majestic and grand. The path through it is cool and dark. Only to step beneath the canopy is to set loose the imagination of child and grandpa alike. The talk was of witches and fear of abandonment. One heard mad cackling laughter and agonized groans. Through at last into the sunlight, we made our way slowly past the fascination of several backhoes, earth-moving vehicles of exotic variety, as well as the common dumptruck. Visited the Princess Tree, a weeping white birch of extraordinary beauty and delicacy. Wrote our names in pen on the white bark, Emmy's a full three inches above last year's. On to the Magic Tree, that monumental weeping beech composed of three massive parts: elephant, dinosaur, crocodile. Extensive climbing carried out, and riding on trunk, tail—whatever member presented itself. Then to the Wizard Walk, a low narrow fence ideal for walking while holding the hand of a grandpa. Many turns back and forth. Homeward bound, stopped to watch the workmen at the Taft (Davies) Mansion, which is now taking on its ancient splendor. Through the Bamboo Forest to the kitchen and a snack.

The visit has been long and excessively tiring, but nonetheless grand, despite the stopping of any inkshed. In a desperate flurry of activity, Jon cemented the crumbling front steps, tamped the driveway with new blacktop, collected specimens of daylilies, etc., to take back to France (illegal, but). On Monday, Jon came to the Boys Friendly lunch, where he was a huge hit. I have now displayed both boys with éclat.

I was accidentally struck in the left eye by a toy thrown by Danny. For three days there has been a dark floater and some dimness of vision. I feel quite kicked out of the world by the discomfort, watery diarrhea, upset stomach, and the usual deadly fatigue. It is amazing that this body has lasted for seventy-one years, considering the odds against survival. It goes contrary to nature somehow. Nothing can be accomplished. The very idea of traveling to Prague, where I'm to speak on "Skin" to the Society of Dermopathology, is terrifying. A great relief to have scotched Budapest and Vienna. I couldn't have made it. Prague alone may just be the overdose that . . .

Bought fruit and vegetables at a Korean market. Greeted the proprietor with a hearty "Jinji jopsu simnikka?" ("Good morning." Literally: "Have you eaten rice today?" Implication: "If so, it has been a good morning.") At which Papa-san summoned the clan of twelve, who gathered about smiling and bowing and jabbering in Korean. With a final "kom-op-sumnidda" (thank you), I was universally understood to be a master of language.

To an ophthalmologist about the dark floaters, the occasional peripheral flash of light, diminished visual acuity, and vague discomfort in the left eye. There is no retinal detachment or injury. The symptoms should all gradually subside. Then came serendipity in the form of a pigmented lesion on the sclera which will have to be biopsied. In the meantime I shall read some books.

In bed at seven-thirty, heavy of heart at having lived so long to so little purpose. A slender girlish moon above. A night of erotic dreaming, myself and the other caparisoned for love.

Tinkered anew with the Rothko. Can't seem to let go of this piece. This will be the third "final version" sent off to the agent. It could be that this is the best of the five art talks. Rothko was looking within himself, without the framework of religion or myth. What he found there was utterly private. He makes no effort to describe or explain. It is so private as to seem on the very edge of chaos. I don't pretend to know what Rothko meant by *No. 3,* I only know that even as you gaze, the painting turns molten. Your eyes and ears fill up with red, your mouth too, so that you see, hear, and taste nothing but red. It has found its way into your veins. You are afloat in it. Frantic, you cast about for some other color, white even, to dilute the intensity, but there is none. You must surrender. The skeptical eye receives this red and wonders at the effrontery of an artist who is so deeply engaged in the meaningless. But it is a tenacious red that will not leave the retina. As the minutes pass, you gaze on until it is no longer a flat painting but a doorway through which you step. Ahead are perspectives of infinity, as though Rothko had summoned into his studio supernatural forces to play upon his brushes. Now and then the waters of the Red Sea part, and you see between the rolling cliffs of crimson a vision. Just as quickly, the vision is drawn back into the canvas, losing its outline, and all that is left is the memory of what had been glimpsed.

Letter from a medical student asking about the meaning of life, death and immortality. I shall do as the Buddha did: lift a lotus flower, smile, and refuse to speak.

Still wrestling with the notion of the tenth book. Only an overreacher would dare it. It goes against Nature somehow. Rilke's tenth Duino Elegy is a big letdown from the nine that precede it. I feel I have already given birth to the child and book no. 10 is just the placenta. Nietzsche said the great secret of life is to die at the right time. The great secret of art is to quit at the right time, as Shakespeare did.

Janet's birthday. Doon and the grandchildren visiting for a week. On Monday, Wednesday, and Friday, I am a child. On Tuesday, Thursday, and Saturday, I am an old man. I have a vision of an old gray man rocking back and forth on a plastic chair in Machine City (the area between Sterling and Cross Campus libraries, which is filled with vending machines). His head is a skull with a candle guttering inside. It is not a pretty sight.

It is curious that to Jon, Larry, and Gretchen, Saint Ronan Terrace is the Earthly Paradise. That in such a stony soil their homely sentiments flourished. Here comes September and the long visits of children and grandchildren continue. For me, the joy of their annual appearance is tinged with fatigue, but for all of them the rapture is undiluted. I shall never do anything to undermine it.

Received the Spanish translation of an early story of mine, "The Consultation," done admirably by Leopoldo Acuna, an M.D. and Ph.D. who is starting a program in Medical Humanities at La Plata Medical School somewhere near Buenos Aires. I shall write to encourage him.

My turn to do the marketing. I went to Ferraro's, my favorite grocery store. It is a bazaar swirling with people of many colors—blacks, Hispanics, Asians, and a majority of Italians. The food is as multicultural as the curriculum at Yale: fish heads, tripe, papayas, veal hearts (for making soffrito). Everything is sold in bulk for feeding large families, every member of which seems always to have come along. The older children push the younger in grocery carts. The women are darkly voluptuous with buttocks of international scope. Their laughter raises the temperature in the market and bedews the produce. I see no ill in the surge in immigration: it lends a place a polyglot vivacity.

Read the Magnificat—Luke 1:46, Mary's canticle in praise of God. She expresses precisely the kind of religious joy that I cannot share. Also, it is smug, self-congratulatory, and wildly class conscious.

Attended the memorial service for a former colleague (hematologist) and acquaintance. Dead at eighty-five after having been incapacitated for five years by a massive stroke. He has been unable to communicate since then. The service was abominable. The rabbi was a young woman who may well have had dyslexia, as she stumbled over every other word. She exuded vulgarity and stupidity. Very pretty, though. The cantor was another woman, this one with a caterwauling sort of soprano and a facial expression last seen on Bernini's *Ecstasy of Saint Theresa*. She gave a hugely irritating rendition of "ayl molay rachamim" and of the Twenty-third Psalm. I reiterated my wishes to Janet that, when the times comes, I don't want there to be any service. Just burnt and scattered, thank you. She nodded unconvincingly.

I am at the Outpatient Surgery Clinic, where I'm to have a pigmented lesion removed from my left eyeball. Coincidentally, this very operating room had been my bedroom all during my internship in 1953. The thought fails to make me feel at home.

"Are you at all vaso-vagal?" the surgeon wants to know.

"Do I faint?"

"Uh-huh. You want it sitting up or lying down?"

"Lying down," I tell him. "It will be like old times." I explain that what had once been the quarters of the house staff had been remodeled as their clinic. "And yes, I can be vaso-vagal, if provoked." I'm invited to assume the table.

Breathes there a man with nerves so dead / That cutting into his eye gives him no dread? It is an elemental fear emphasized by the fact that you can watch the blade descending. Your eyelids are being held open by a metal retractor. The natural recoil of blinking has been taken away from you. The idea of an anesthetic being injected into your eye is only the beginning. There comes the sound of the snipping of scissors. "Snip, snip, snip." It is the cruelest sound of your life. You imagine aqueous humor and blood running down your cheek. You think of poor Gloucester thus enucleated by Cornwall in act 3 of *King Lear* and of Cornwall's postoperative exclamation. You decide to say it aloud.

"Out vile jelly! Where is thy lustre now?" The surgeon pauses in his infernal snipping. He is aghast.

"Why did you say that?" Even his voice is pale. Ah, the power of language that can set a mighty surgeon's hand atremble. Now it is he who is distinctly vaso-vagal. I should have waited until he finished.

※

Prague: it is a city suspended from the five hundred spires that are its only skyscrapers. A thousand years of religious ardor—Catholic, Protestant, Jewish—add to the sense of being aloft, on high. The odor of sanctity and the odor of sewage, blended, is what you inhale here. God and shit are inseparable in the lungs of the Czech Republic.

We have seen a good deal more than I had hoped—a deadly round of sightseeing and concerts (Mozart lived here). I prefer minimalism: to see one sight, the greatest one, and keep it in the deepest chamber of my mind. As it is, Prague is a blur, out of focus. But I am not a free man, and am practiced in the arts of placation, congeniality, and obedience. Still, Prague is worthy of the praise heaped upon it. Not even the army of tourists can rub out the beauty of Prague. I saw the house where Kafka was born, and one he lived in. Rilke lived here too. But me? I'm counting the hours until I get back to New Haven. I'd feel same after a week in Heaven.

The Czech people are so good-looking. Both men and women are slim, with superb upholstery, blond hair, and good teeth. Next to a Czech I am a misbegotten dwarf, a Quasimodo, someone who would do the world a kindness by keeping covered head to toe and sitting in dark corners. Prague is death on one's self-esteem. I have seen no more than half a dozen children, so the populace has apparently gotten birth control down pat.

The talk that I gave was intended for the International Society of Dermatopathology, but it was delivered to an empty hall, as three-quarters of the doctors got up and left while I was being introduced, and the rest, save for a few of the timid, walked out within the first five minutes. Nevertheless I soldiered on and was presented with a plaque which gave my name as Robert Selzer and spelled Prague with a *q* instead of a *g*: *Praque*. But let me not whine. We must pray for those who do not understand us.

Janet has had a splendid time what with flying first class, a Jacuzzi in the hotel room, me to boss around, and ten thousand things to buy. I may have to go on the literary dole after this. I'll be home Tuesday night—forty-eight hours from right now. Strike up the band!

Home from Prague at two this morning, convinced that I shall not go anywhere ever again. Not that there is anywhere that can match the matchless: the city is magical—there but not there, palpable but elusive, like the corpse of a beautiful woman whose flesh can still be touched but whose persona is no more—it endures only in either memory or imagination. But the horrors of velocity are too much for me. I am not comfortable in the crotch of a taut rubber band being shot from one continent to the other. From now on, *you* go. I'm staying here.

I had invited Janet to come along, intent that she enjoy a fine time. And so she did until I lost the case holding the grandchildren's presents, her souvenirs, et cetera. Lost it irretrievably somewhere in the locale of the Detroit airport baggage area. Yes, Detroit. Doesn't everyone come home from Prague via Detroit? So I have once again learned that Hell is paved with good intentions. *Carramba!*

Home to the news that my dearest high school chum has died suddenly in Troy. I'll drive up and back on Friday for the funeral. Can't have him lowered into the Trojan earth behind my back, now, can I?

I'm reading a collection of vignettes by a young surgeon, Frank Hroyler —wonderful. No need to look over my shoulder to see who's gaining on me. This guy, in one stunning dash, and *with* stunning dash, has caught up and passed me. I'll drizzle dressing on it in the *San Francisco Chronicle* with the pleasure of benediction and the pain of being surpassed. Toss me onto the trash heap of Chronos—I'm ready.

Friday I drove up to Troy for the funeral of my dearest high school chum. We were fourteen together, then fifteen, sixteen, and eighteen. The sweetest time of life and the most excruciating. I have loved him for half a century. Arrived at ten o'clock, parked only a block from the house of my youth, climbed the seventy-two white granite steps called the Approach to 8th Street, walked north on a street with no sidewalks, past vacancy and dilapidation, passed Federal, People's, and Jacob Streets. At Eagle turned right, up the steep hill to 9th where, at the corner of Eagle and 9th, stands the Armenian Apostolic Church. Henry Tutunjian lay there in a coffin draped with an American flag—he was a judge. The sight of that box and the knowledge of the treasure it held weakened my resolve, but I didn't cry until the "Soorp Soorp" (Holy Holy) from the Armenian liturgy. We all recited the Lord's Prayer in Armenian. "Hyer Mer" is "Our Father." It had been written out phonetically for us heathens to join in. "Down, Troy!" I cried. "You'll have your bone!" Such is a walk in that lethargic exhausted town: up a grand classical staircase, down streets of decay and neglect to stand before the corpse of the beloved. The drive back to New Haven was slow and consolatory, with the leaves turning. Nature doesn't let you grieve for long.

Home from Prague for a week and still my mind is filled with mystical visions. The place surely does have "eine mystische gestalt"—Kafka was right. From dawn to midnight we strolled—the flâneries of the tourist—ate and drank in catacombs below narrow streets where every doorknocker is a masterpiece of arabesque ironwork. Outside the hotel on Wenceslas Square an all-night rampage of youth—song, laughter, dancing, drumbeats. No one sleeps in Prague. Then—what's this? A few dozen white-clad shaven-headed Hare Krishnas jingle by, to say nothing of the hourly, half-hourly, and quarter-hourly bells and the carts of the streetcleaners.

A Tale of Two Cities, then: Prague and Troy. It would take Dickens to depict them fairly. I have written about Troy the way Czechs have written about Prague—with the same nostalgia, a blend of love and hate. Between pragueness and trojaneity, give me my own native land. In Troy I am of the blood; in Prague I was a temporary graft.

Sitting at a table in the Sterling, I am asked by a student if I will tie his necktie. A glance reveals the absence of hands. Thalidomide? He has a faint German accent and my mother's eyes—soft, moist, and brown. I stand behind him, uncertain and shaky. There is nothing of the surgeon's self-assurance in my hands, the way they fumble. The act is one of great intimacy. I feel his breath upon my hands, my wrist rests upon his neck. The boy's utter submission. At last it is done. I move the knot under his chin and button the shirt beneath it.

"I have an interview today," he tells me.

"Then you need to look your best. Good luck."

Asked the young pharmacist at the drugstore for four ounces of glycerine and rose water.

"For what?"

"For my chapped hands."

"Never heard of it."

"Well, then," and I walked haughtily away. By just such pitiful jeux d'esprits do I try to keep going on.

Last evening at the Medical School, a highly charged theatrical performance by a pediatric hematologist on the subject of "The Marriage of Art and Science." Who would have thought the doctor to have had so much ham in him? And all delivered in a plummy British accent about which he made much. He opened and closed with two overwrought, sentimental poems about the death of his child-patients, each of which would have made slapstick of Little Nell. Nothing could have been more maudlin, calculating, or hypocritical. His thesis, I believe, is that the arts have a healing effect. He urges everyone in the profession to write poems. Then, too, we must not take ourselves too seriously. He himself wears false noses, wigs, funny socks, and ties to work—a regular clown. The jewel in the crown of his address was this:

He was asked by the parents of an eight-year-old boy dying of leukemia to tell the boy the truth in order that there be no "conspiracy of silence" among them. The scene is set meticulously. Mother and child sit side by side on the couch in his cluttered office, the floor of which is strewn with papers and toys. The father leans against a door. There is a nurse in the room. The doctor sits at his desk (perhaps he is wearing a rubber nose) and says to the boy: "You are going to die and go to Heaven." Quite understandably the boy buries his face in his mother's "yellow" dress and howls for a full three minutes while the four adults weep openly. After three minutes, the boy abruptly quietens, looks about at the clutter, and speaks: "Didn't your mother ever teach you to straighten your room?" All at once there is laughter, healing. The mood changes from terror and despair to relief.

But who was healed here? Certainly not the boy and his parents. It is the doctor who, with his false nose and loud socks and devotion to candor, has made himself feel better. A disgusting display of self-absorption. It is cruelty in the garb of candor. If I know anything about myself, I know that I could never tell an eight-year-old boy that he will die and go to Heaven. I haven't the bone marrow for it.

Lunched alone at the hospital cafeteria. It has by far the most interesting clientele in the city, what with the quantities of chromosomal patrons.

Today there were eight of the elvish, the hunchbacked, the scarce-half-made-up—the unfinished, as Richard III has it. Add to that the massively obese, the emaciated, a man with alopecia totalis, a wrinkled and stooped young woman with progeria, and you have a full plate of fascination to go with your soup and sandwich.

⟊

Outside Mory's, a small tree, hardly more than a shrub, with some two dozen dry brown leaflets waggling still and a dozen brown sparrows indistinguishable from the leaves by shade or motion. One lifts a wing and could just as well be a leaf fluttering. A leaf flaps and could be a bird. They are perfectly camouflaged, and so are quite willing to ignore an umbrella tapping the trunk of the tree.

⟊

This morning I mounted to the summit of East Rock, my substitute for a Sunday sermon. It was sunny and cool with a brisk December wind. From there I went to Evergreen Woods for a visit with Maynard, who is in and out of his mind. I found him in better spirits, though still obsessed with a desire to go home. I read to him from the diary of Samuel Pepys. When he laughed it did my heart good. His wife, Florence, has hired two graduate students to come out twice a week and read to him. He loves it and takes immense pleasure in reciting the next line before the student can read it. When he related this, I swung my hat and shouted, Hallelujah! I believe his mood may be lighter, but it could be illusory. To live for a day at ninety is damn hard work.

⟊

Spent a couple, three days just hangin' round waitin' for the Millennium, writing only letters and reading a biography of Mark Twain. Terribly sad to learn that the man who amused millions was despondent for the latter part of his life. Beloved wife dead, one daughter dead of "brain fever," another with uncontrolled epilepsy. And bankrupt after investing all his money in a kind of printing machine. Interesting that he stage-managed his career down to the last detail, e.g., those white suits for which he earned the sobriquet the Whited Sepulchre. Once, having been invited to give a presentation along with James Whitcomb Riley, he accepted on condition that Riley would eschew all humor and take the serious tack only—he didn't want any rivals. Then he proceeded to memorize all of his material so that he could talk without notes. What a far cry from my own shabby behavior at the podium. My heart goes out to Mark Twain, a truly lovable character.

I was daydreaming in the Sterling when a vagrant thought found its way out of my head to materialize magnified before my eyes. Must have slipped through a foramen or a small separation in a suture line of the skull—the coronal, say, or the sagittal—and from there through a pore of the scalp left ajar. It was a cloud the size and shape of a football, with a single drop of blood at the center. I knew at once that it is the murder I have imagined committing again and again. I reached out to grasp it but my hand passed right through, back and forth. When I withdrew, there was her blood on my fingers.

The thought occurs that one is saved by one's ordinariness. The shallower the man, the more durable he is and the more he can endure. That is the way it is with me. Had I been deeper, more introspective, more intellectually honest, more moral; had I been a man with feelings deeper than a teary sentimentality, I should have long since collapsed under the bombardment of life. I have a vision of myself sitting in a dark corner. I moan, then get up and go to a window, clutch a handful of the curtain, draw it back, and peer into the blackness of night—it would always be night—then return to the corner and moan again. That is what I might have done if . . . But as it is, I blithely bathe and dress the wounds that eat their way to the surface. By tomorrow they'll have scabbed over. The blackness that had hung over my eyes and invaded my body is not there in the morning. The sun is shining. It is well that self-loathing doesn't show on one's face.

The library will be closed for three days. I shall have delirium tremens by Sunday noon. I've half a mind to lie down on the floor of my carrel, lights out, and stay snug until Monday. I know the place down to the last alcove and can get to the toilet, coffee machine, and Tampax dispenser in the dark. What else do I need? I have that last article in mind, Tampax, as this morning Janet informed me that my granddaughter has started menstruating. She is not ready for it. I am not ready for it either. *Turn back, turn back, O time in thy flight* . . . And with the library closed too! There is the scent of Millennium in the air. Next thing you know—*poof.* Funny thing about shutting down one's haunts (the gym too is locked): there are suddenly buckets of time, the kind that doesn't pass, but stands still. You look at the clock. It says ten to one. An hour later you look again. It's still ten to one. The time is out of joint, all right.

Read Matisse's account of Renoir at work. It seems that Renoir suffered from an extreme form of arthritis. All of his joints were frozen. In addition, he had numerous ulcerations, abscesses, and open, bleeding sores. He had to hold the brush between thumb and forefinger, and high up in the first web space. An assistant would move the canvas according to his direction. All the life was in Renoir's eyes, which were clear and alert. And that one bloody paw. The rest was almost dead. Still he refused to quit and went on working until the last breath. The painting was of a beautiful young girl, full of health and life. What could have been the diagnosis? Scleroderma? Dermatomyositis? Rheumatoid arthritis with secondary infections? I must try to find out.

Last night, a phone call from Mad J. no. 2, largely incoherent due to the tachyphemia. He called from the mental hospital where he has been for three weeks.

"Why are you there this time?"

"I was decompensating."

He is "terribly lonely," implores me to visit him.

"(*Gently.*) No, I cannot do that. Are you at least physically comfortable?"

"I am comfortably miserable."

He is taking seven medications but refuses to take the antipsychotic medication Haldol.

"Why?"

"It prevents ejaculation."

He told me of the month he spent with a family at the foot of West Rock. It was the happiest month of his life, and every morning he was treated to the rising of the sun over the Rock. "So beautiful." We wish each other a Happy New Year. I cannot fall asleep for the pity of it. And the guilt. But I know better than to visit him.

Janet and Becky left for France on a ten-day visit with Jon. I shall let moss grow over my brain and see no one, if I can help it. Still I shall keep on polishing paragraphs, stitching words into sentences. It gives me something to do, and I love to do it. Yale University is celebrating the birth of Jesus by keeping everyone out of its buildings, all of which are locked and bolted. This includes the library, gym, computer cluster, and every other of my lairs. In desperation I took myself down to the Medical School on the assumption that it would have been exempt. Suppose a doctor had to look up the directions for some procedure—version and breech extraction, say, with the poor woman in hard labor and the baby lying wrong way up, and the door to the Medical Library locked? Grounds for malpractice, I'd say.

With the survival instincts of the homeless, I gave the guard my most brilliant smile and sailed on down a corridor of laboratories, then up one flight through a door marked "Keep Out," down another flight, and found myself in a lovely small amphitheater, a replica of one of those nineteenth-century lecture halls, only tiny. There are only four tiers, no more than thirty-five seats altogether. Between rows 2 and 3, and 3 and 4, there are two stairs to climb, so that the room is raked steeply. The floors and seats are of light-colored wood, the railings, fixtures, and walls of Yale blue. On the blackboard in large cursive letters someone had written the word *Surgery* followed by an exclamation point. I felt welcome in what then and there became a hallowed place. It was in this very amphitheater that I once gave a reading from *Down from Troy*. I believe I even sang "Mexicali Rose," thereby shocking the august faculty. That was ten or more years ago, and I haven't seen the room since. With immense pleasure I sat down and spent two hours of sheltered obscurity until it was time to hunt for lunch.

2000

FOR ALL MY STUDY OF SCIENCE, I half believe that every rock, pool, tree, flame, cloud, and crag contains a presence that has a certain awareness. It's what comes of being an old cracked beaker of Russian, Hebrew, and Celtic blood. Even as a doctor I would place my stethoscope on an elderly chest and hear the beat of Psyche's wings. It is a longing for the lost primitive link to the earth. In my life, I am an average man and I am a pagan. I strive to be good-natured and decent, never to be saintly. I don't care about pleasing God, only Man. Banned from the place where love occurs, I have tried, first through surgery, then through writing, to find the meaning of human existence and to place myself in a creative relationship with it.

Years ago as a doctor and more recently as a writer, I declared my faith in images—the human fact placed near a superhuman mystery, even if both are illusions of the senses. Diagnosis, like writing, calls for the imagination and the skill to discover things not seen, things that hide themselves under the shadow of natural objects. It is the purpose of the writer and the doctor to fix these unseen phenomena in words, thereby presenting to plain sight what did not actually exist until he arrived, much as a footprint hides beneath a foot until a step is taken.

Bamboo is the irresistible demonic force before which man is humbled. Today I counted more than a hundred new canes of it in the patch Jon planted a quarter of a century ago, each one furious to be born into the upper air, as angry as any infant half in and half out of the birth canal and squeezed by the contractions of womb and pelvic musculature alike. It will not be denied, the way it upthrusts through piles of brush and dead leaves and turns aside rocks in the rage to live. Here is bamboo as lumber, as fully armed warrior sprung from a seed. Here is the god Bamboo.

To the pathologist, the grand implication of an autopsy is of abounding life to come. The dissector in the morgue rummages in this hotel of bones, with its arterial corridors, thoracic lobbies, and windows curtained with membrane, searching for the legacy of the newly dead. He is the deliverer of wisdom. Studying and dissecting the human body, far from desacralizing it, increases its holiness. Leonardo da Vinci transformed his knowledge of the body into a transcendental art; the medical student transforms it into the power to heal.

As for harvesting the human heart, it is no recent innovation. It was on one of the Crusades that the Sire de Courcy, mortally wounded in battle with the Turk, bade his servant cut out his heart and carry it back to the Dame de Fayel, whom he had long and ardently loved. It happened that her husband intercepted the gift and had it cooked into a "well-relished" dish. This he compelled his wife to eat, assuring her that it was a "cordial for her weakness." Once she had eaten it all, he told her the truth, whereupon in a "sudden exaltation of joy" she gave a "far-fetch'd sigh" and licked the platter clean. In the morning she was found dead in her bed.

There was a female patient of mine who felt, as I do, that the flesh and the spirit are one and the same thing, that the flesh is the spirit thickened. From this, she had developed a morbid fear of X-rays. Before I was aware of this, I had ordered a chest X-ray in full exhalation. "Take a deep breath. Blow it all out. Now *hold* it," said the technician from behind his lead shield. The woman knew at once that what she had blown out on command was not just air, it was a part of her that mattered, her soul. At first she hadn't dared to tell me that it was my fault. When at last she did, she was relieved.

I have just left the Yale Art Gallery, where I have been looking at a painting by Francisco de Zurbarán. It shows Mary and Jesus at home in Nazareth. The teenage Jesus, dressed in a pale lavender tunic and bare-foot, has been weaving a circlet of thorns and has just pricked his finger. He bends to examine his wound, his face nearly touching his hand. Mary, dressed in a voluminous scarlet robe, has paused in her sewing and is contemplating the boy with a tender look of infinite sadness, as if she has foreknowledge of what is to come. The entire scene is still, motionless, otherworldly, mystical. This despite such homely details as a large basket of white laundry on the floor, some pears on a table whose drawer is partially open, a vase of flowers. A shaft of celestial light descends on the room. In it one sees cherubim treading air and looking down at the mother and son. While the boy is engrossed in his wounded finger, the mother's attention is upon her son to the exclusion of all else. At the bottom of the picture, two plump white doves gaze directly outward, as though acknowledging the presence of the viewer.

Outside the Art Gallery there is a row of low stone benches attached to the front of the building. On the last of these a black man and woman sit, so close together as to seem engrafted the one upon the other. Her left hand emerges from beneath his right arm. Their heads are pressed together at the temples. Passing by, I overhear a bit of dialogue:

SHE: I love you more than you love me.
HE: You can't possibly love me more than I love you.
SHE: Yes, I do.
HE: No, you don't.
SHE: Yes, I do.

I had already turned the corner from Chapel into High Street, but now I reverse my steps until I can observe them. She is the older, but by how much it is at first difficult to tell. She is wearing a woolen cap that

covers her hair, and a shapeless, bulky overcoat. Aside from a few stream-
lets of oysterish, barely pigmented cloud, the sky is deeply blue. I stop to
talk. It's that kind of day, noontime after all, when both hands of the clock
are lifted in either supplication or hallelujah. All about them, on the
cobblestones, pigeons are billing.

ME: Are you lovers?
SHE: Yes we' lovers. He' my son. I love him to death.
ME: Do you love him more than he loves you?
SHE: Yes, I do.
HE: No, you don't.
SHE: Yes, I do.
ME: Are you having a fight?
SHE: Yes, this is the way we fight.

The woman is perhaps fifty, with a broad, somewhat tipsy grin, her
speech a little slurred. She is smoking a cigarette.

SHE: Come on over here, man, and give me a shake.

She holds out her hand. I take it in mine. It is soft and dry. She raises
my hand to her lips, kisses it. Her breath, too, is a warm dry softness.
When she smiles I see that she has only two mandibular teeth so widely
spaced as to be useless for chewing. He is in his thirties, I decide, with a
small black moustache, a gold necklace and ring, a baseball cap, tracksuit
pants and jacket, and large running shoes. There is a bandage on his right
index finger.

ME: How did you hurt your finger?
HE: Pullin' up a dead rose bush at her house.

Now they resume their argument over the relative intensity of their
love for each other. I cannot be sure, but I think that my presence has

spurred them on to even more vehemence in their tender reproaches. That is the effect of an audience on the players.

ME: You're the luckiest people in the city.
HE: We know it. We know it, don't we?
SHE: Uh-huh, we do.

For a long time I stand somewhere between her saying "I love you more," and his denying it. Theirs is a unique happiness with its own wisdom. But happiness is too unlucky to last. It will end violently. See how she turns to gaze at his left ear, studying the delicate whorl of cartilage, reaching to touch the earlobe that is as soft as love itself. I want to warn her but I can't speak. Besides, it wouldn't do any good. *Die now!* I want to say. Only you go first this time. I shiver in their warmth and listen to my teeth chattering. I can smell their suffering.

Could such a scene have been received between mere eyelids, these two sitting on the bench, pressed into each other? The smoke from her cigarette encloses him in a uterine mantle. At the outer edge, New Haven itself is smoky, elastic, elusive. It seems to me that the *sitzgruppe* has risen off the ground. I have to look up to see them atop the pedestals upon which they have placed each other, where they are blurred as in a celestial astigmatism. Above them pigeons, plump and weightless, have gathered on a ledge. From beneath each lifted wing, light is released. They might be cherubim giving off incense and effulgence and music. It is well known that the senses of cherubim are not distinct but blend and flow into one another in a kind of angelic synesthesia. What is that smell? Sandalwood, I think, or frankincense.

It is absurd, this kneeling down inside my soul. But already I have heated ink, dipped a scalpel, and carved a tear on my left cheek. It burns all the way down. The mother smiles, and there again are the two canine teeth.

"Open your mouth, Mother. This won't hurt. They're so loose. They waggle. There! It's done. Rinse with this. Now spit."

Teeth of the Virgin . . . wrapped in velvet and resting in a tiny reliquary of gold and lapis lazuli. Harvested and donated anonymously to the Yale Art Gallery, where a river of adoring gazes will bathe them from now on, wearing them thin and translucent and all the holier for it.

I walk away. They remain, telling on, one bead after another in contrapuntal argument, until the whole chain will have been recited, then begun anew. Hushed are the pigeons on the high ledges. Only when I have turned the corner do they resume their cooing until, as at a sign, they flutter up, wings whirring, and escort me away. Blessed are the people who sit on benches in the city. Blessed are the mother and her son. In the middle of the block on High Street, I tumble headlong to the pavement in a pool of words . . .

Time and again, I have returned to the corner of Chapel and High to stand by the stone bench, now vacant, straining to see departed splendor. Sometimes I remove my glasses and gaze into the city's dust, turned golden by the sun, and I have the faint sense that here in this place are things not ready to be seen. The full significance of the encounter lies in its echo, which only I was privileged to hear. For a brief moment, eternity became visible . . . palpable . . . audible . . . when, beneath a noonday sun, a stone bench occupied by two persons became an imperishable vision to which I am bound by invisible chains. It seems to me now that mother and son had been waiting there for my participation, the way a blank mirror waits for the image it is meant to reflect.

Let me be at that place by the gallery.

Let the noonday sun be warm and bright.

Let there be sitting a woman and a youth.

Let him be weaving a crown of thorns.

Let him prick his finger, then bend to examine the wound.

Let her be dressed in a scarlet gown.

Let him wear a tunic of pale lavender.

Let him be barefoot.

Let there be a basket of white linen by her feet.

Let her be sewing.

Let her gaze at him with tenderness and sorrow.

Let her reach out to touch the lobe of his ear.
Let her feel its softness as a wound in her heart.
Let me feel her beatific breath upon my hand.
Let there be doves on the ledge above them.
Let the bench live inside me.
Let me keep it there.

Since I am no longer a writer, I have decided to become a lover. But to whom shall I make advances? To *what* would be more optimistic. A person of my slackness and saccularity cannot afford to set limitations. Perhaps I should lie down and take a nap.

In the election, 6 Saint Ronan Terrace continues to buck the tide. The country went its own self-destructive way. The coming apocalypse will not be our fault. At the polling station (or whatever it's called) the registrar (or whatever you call her) asked to see my photo ID, "even though you fixed my hernia." I told her I'd show her my ID if she showed me her incision. End of sally.

Haiku
treelet
beetles faint and recover
gone all harmony and meaning
no streetlamps hanging in the fog

Persephone returns each year from Hell as springtime, quickening the life within the seed, warming the cool bud with her breath. It is fitting that

Persephone is always seen in art and literature as a girl embodied in a tree, a plant, a flower. Ezra Pound: "The milk-white girls / Unbend from the holly-trees."

Perhaps the strangest achievement of biotechnology has been to re-enact the myth of Persephone, to make the mythic real. There is the ever-present notion of harvest and transplantation, of renewal. The rebirth, the springtime, exists in the new life of the heart recipient. Persephone is once again the goddess of metamorphosis, with the power to grow toward rejuvenation. Hers is the promise of rebirth out of the dark.

Time was, when a youth was sacrificed to bring on an early spring or to ensure a good harvest. The killing was carried out with all due solemnity and in accordance with ritual. There was the flash of a blade. A flag of blood unfurled from the youth's neck. It was understood by the others, and even by the youth, that this was good to do. It was pro bono publico. Perhaps the "victim" prayed to be chosen. There was glory in the occasion. One rose to it willingly. But that was long ago.

At 2:30 a woman stepped up to the desk where I was sitting. "Dr. Selzer?" She had driven down from Saratoga to talk about dialogue in the writing of memoir. Weeks ago I had said yes, she could come, but neglected to write it down and forgot. The dear, sweet security guards, who all cover up for me, came to find me for her and made it all better. I spent an hour with her, in which I caused her to fall in love with me. I tell you, the combination of being adorable and an icon is no cinch.

Conversation with six-year-old Emmy:

"Is it true, Grandpa, that when you were a boy, you had a pet stegosaurus?"

"Oh, yes indeed."

"I don't entirely believe you."

"I remember the feel of it—cold and scaly. No fur."

"I know they don't have any fur!"

"It was a baby stegosaurus. The spines were small and not sharp, still soft. It didn't eat people or any other animal. Only grass and . . ."

"Salad?"

"Yes, salad. A lot of salad. I had to take it for a walk three times a day. On a leash."

"Did you take it outside to go to the bathroom?"

"No. Just for a walk. It didn't make any duty. Just every once in a while a few lavender bubbles came out."

"What else?"

"I'd take it up through the Bamboo Forest in back of the house and all the way to the Magic Tree where it would climb up on a branch and take a nap while I rocked it up and down."

"Oh Grandpa! I want to have a pet stegosaurus too!"

The reader will see the diabolically clever way in which Grandpa ignores the little girl's disbelief and proceeds at once to the details of skin, scales, spines, diet, and, above all, bowel movements. Grandpa is well aware that to a six-year-old, there is nothing more riveting than matters excremental. The reader will notice at precisely what point the child willingly suspended her disbelief and was taken prisoner by her grandpa. (*Wild maniacal laughter!*)

A writer ought not to expect or desire that his wife or partner read his work and offer comment. Nothing could be more harmful to a marriage. Let us abide with one another on other terms.

JANET: What are you smiling about?

ME: I assure you it is against the grain.

He is the sort of birdwatcher who leaps out from behind a bush, blocks your path and proceeds to wax statistical as to the great number and rarity of the birds he has seen in this very spot not more than an hour ago, but which, alas, seem to have moved on, as they aren't there now. This last delivered with a tiny rueful smile.

The way she put out her hand, fingering the darkness, feeling the nap of it.

Accosted by another retired surgeon who bent close and told me in a low, furtive voice about his research. He adds carcinogenic substances to the feed of laboratory rats, waits a period of time, then colonoscopes the rats looking for polyps. Surely this must be done at some risk to one's point of view? I so expressed myself. His melancholy smile told me that the damage had already been done. I too fell into a conspiratorial mode. "Perhaps," I said, "it might help to think of the body as a church occupied by a congregation of organs of which the mightiest is the heart. Even from the rectum of a rat, one might listen for the sound of the Great Amen."

Some reflections on pain. "Why do you write so much about pain?" they ask me. *To give it a name,* I reply, and I am not sure what I mean. I try again: in October, when the leaves have fallen from the trees, you can see farther into the forest. Well . . .

Pain . . . Pain is fire, a ravening, insatiable thing that insists upon utter domination. It is the occasion when the body reasserts itself over the mind. The universe contracts about the part that hurts. If the pain is not placated with analgesics, it will devour the whole organism. Only then will it, too, be snuffed. Still, pain is revelatory. In the blaze of it one might catch a glimpse of the truth about human existence.

It was the poet Rilke who wrote that the events of the body cannot be rendered in language. Surely this is so with pain as with its opposite, orgasm. These extremes of sensation remain beyond the power of language to express. Say that a doctor is examining a patient who is in pain. The doctor needs to know the exact location of the pain and its nature. Is the pain sharp or dull? Steady or intermittent? Does it throb or pulse? Is it stabbing? A heavy pressure? Crampy? Does it burn? Sting? But there is no wholly adequate way for the sufferer to portray his pain, other than to cry out. The patient, like the writer, must resort to metaphor, simile, imagery—"It's as if someone were digging in my ribs with a shovel," "Feels as if there's a heavy rock on my chest"—to bring the doctor to a partial understanding of his pain. In order to express it fully, he would have to cry out in a language that is incomprehensible to anyone else. This language of pain has no consonants, but consists only of vowels— *ow! aiee! oy! oh!*—punctuated by grunts, sobs, moans, gasps. It is a self-absorbed language that might have been the first ever uttered by prehistoric man. Perhaps it was learned from animals. These howled vowels have the eloquence of the wild, the uncivilized, the atavistic. Comprehension is instantaneous, despite the absence of what we call words. It is a mode of expression beyond normal language. Nor could it be made more passionate or revelatory by the most gifted writer, not even Shakespeare.

But what is the purpose of these cries of pain? Wouldn't silence be as eloquent? For one thing, the loud, unrestrained pouring forth of vowels is useful for attracting the attention of anyone within earshot who might come to the assistance of the sufferer. Vowels carry farther than consonants and are easier to mouth, requiring only the widely opened jaws, without the more complex involvement of tongue, teeth, and palate that consonants demand. Verdi knew this and made his librettist write lines full of easily singable vowels and diphthongs. It is the sung vowel that carries to the last row of La Scala. The consonants are often elided or faked by the singers, who know that consonants are confined to the immediate vicinity of the stage and are altogether less able to be infused with emotive force. It comes as no surprise that the greatest operas are in the Italian repertoire—Italian, a language dripping with vowels, in which there is scarcely a word that does not end in one. "Mille serpi divoranmi il petto," sings the anguished Alfredo upon learning of the sacrifice made by his beloved Violetta in *La Traviata*. The translation—"A thousand snakes are eating my breast"—simply won't do.

One purpose of these cries of pain, then, might be to summon help, to notify fellow members of the tribe of one's predicament so that they will come running. But I think there is more to it than that. For the sufferer, these outcries have a kind of magical property of their own, offering not only an outlet for the emotion but a means of letting out the pain. Hollering, all by itself, gives a measure of relief. To cry out *ow!* or *aiee!* requires that the noise be carried away from the body on a cloud of warm, humid air that had been within the lungs of the sufferer. The expulsion of this air, and with it the sound, is an attempt to exteriorize the pain, to dispossess oneself of it, as though the vowels of pain were in some magical way the pain itself. It is not hard to see why the medieval church came to believe that a body writhing, racked, and uttering unearthly, primitive cries was possessed by devils. Faced with such a sufferer, authorities of the church deemed exorcism both necessary and compassionate. "Go ahead and holler," says the nurse to the patient. "You'll feel better. Don't hold it in." It is wise advice that has been passed down through millennia of human suffering.

But even these ululations cannot really convey to the reader what the sufferer is feeling, for they are not literature. To write *ow* or *aiee* on a page is not art. The language of pain, then, is the most exclusive of tongues, spoken and understood by an elite of one. Hearing it, we shudder out of sympathy for the sufferer, but just as much out of the premonition that each of us shall know this language in our time. Our turn will come. It is a fact that within moments of having been relieved of their pain, sufferers are no longer fluent in its language. They have already forgotten it, all but an inkling or two, and are left with a vague sense of dread, a recollection that the pain was awful, a fear that it might return.

In lieu of language, the doctor seems to diagnose by examining the body and its secretions—urine, blood, spinal fluid—and by using a number of ingenious photographic instruments. A last resort would be the laying open of the body for exploratory surgery. Fifty years ago it was to the corpse that the doctor went for answers. Ironic that life should have provided concealment and death be revelatory. Even now it is only in the autopsy room that the true courage of the human body is apparent, the way it carries on in the face of all odds: arteriosclerosis, calculi, pulmonary fibrosis, softening of the brain. And still the body goes on day after day, bearing its burdens if not jauntily, at least with acceptance and obedience, until at last it must come to the morgue, where its faithfulness can be observed and granted homage.

My Iraqi friend Saad Ahmed practices meditation in accordance with an ancient Tibetan text. This is done, he tells me, by focusing on a single object so as to achieve one-mindedness. The spine must be held absolutely straight because of the *chakra*s, those points along the vertebral column that are the seat of disease. Saad says it is possible to negate pain by concentrating on it with extreme intensity. Certainly there is about pain that which exhilarates even as it appalls, as Emily Dickinson has written. Pain is the expression of the dark underside of the body. As such, the sight of the wound and the sound of the outcry it produces stir the imagination in a way that pleasure never can. We are drawn to the vicinity of pain by the hint of danger and death as much as by the desire to compare our fortunate state to that of the sufferer. Then, too, there is the undeniable relation of pain and beauty, brought to artistic flower during the Renaissance and later by the Romantic poets.

It is the writhen Christ slumping on the cross that is the emblematic vision of pain, from which has come the word *excruciating*. In the beginning—I'd bet on it—pain was to be avoided at all costs. Somewhere along the way a harsh, usurpative Christianity commandeered pain and tried to wrest meaning from it, holding it up as the avenue to Paradise. Throughout my childhood I listened to nuns suggesting that I offer up whatever was hurting, either physically or mentally, as if suffering, boredom, or even annoyance were currency to be paid on the road to sanctity. According to Milton, even Satan is not outside the precincts of pain. In the titanic single combat between Satan and the Archangel Michael, the sword of Michael "shear'd / all his right side; then Satan first knew pain." Simone Weil turned affliction into evidence of God's tenderness. Affliction is love, she wrote. To some, this represents a perversion of the senses, not unlike the masochism that welcomes pain as pleasure. To welcome pain as an approach to God is to negate mercy as the proof of his love for human beings. It is an elite band of saints that can achieve ecstasy through pain. Even Christ cried out from the cross, *Why hast thou forsaken me?*

The artist who would prettify or soften the Crucifixion is missing the point. The aim was to kill horribly and to subject the victim to the utmost humiliation. It involved a preliminary whipping with the dreaded Roman *flagrum,* a leather whip with three tails. At the tip of each tail there was tied a small dumbbell-shaped weight of iron or bone. With each lash of the whip, the three bits dug into the flesh. The victim was tied or chained to a post and two centurions stood on either side. The wounds extended around to the chest and abdomen. Profuse bleeding ensued. Then the condemned was beaten on the face with reeds so that his face was bruised, his nose broken. To ensure maximum humiliation, the cross was set up in a public place or on an elevation of land, such as the hill of Calvary. In the case of Jesus, in order to deride him further and to mock his appellation of King of the Jews, a crown of thorns was placed on his brow. Jesus, weakened by a night of fasting and prayer as well as by the flogging and blood loss, was not able to carry his own cross to the place of execution as the punishment required. Simon of Cyrene did it for him. Then Jesus' hands were nailed to the crosspiece, which was raised and set into a groove on the vertical piece. The height was approximately seven and a half feet. At one point, a Roman soldier hurled a spear that opened a wound in his side. To add to Christ's suffering, he was assailed by extreme thirst, as is usual in instances of severe blood loss and dehydration. Once he called for a drink and an onlooker offered him vinegar through a hollow straw. Death came slowly from shock, both traumatic and hypovolemic, and from respiratory failure owing to the difficulty of expelling air from the lungs in the upright and suspended position, in which the diaphragm does not easily rise.

I wonder whether we have not lost the ability to withstand pain, what with the proliferation of pain-killing drugs and anesthetic agents. Physical pain has become a once-in-a-while experience for most of the industrialized world. Resistance to pain, like any other unused talent, atrophies, leaving one all the more vulnerable. What to a woman of the late nineteenth century might have been bearable is insupportable to her great-great-granddaughter. Still, for some, chronic pain is an old adversary, one whose cunning can be, if not negated, at least balanced by hypnosis, acupuncture, biofeedback, exercise, practice of ritual, and other techniques not well understood. Then there is that pain which cannot be relieved by any means short of death and which must be lived *against*. Such was the pain of Montaigne, who, tortured by bladder stones that occluded the outflow of urine, had to write against the pain. In contrast, Aristotle was unable to philosophize because of his toothache.

Is the pain experienced in a dream any less than the so-called real pain experienced while awake? I think it is not. I have a dream that has recurred many times in which I am standing alone in the middle of a great empty amphitheater. It is midnight, and the scene is bathed in bluish moonlight. The city is European: Milan, I think. At either end of the amphitheater a statue stands upon a marble pedestal. One is of Caesar wearing a toga and holding up a sheaf of wheat, the other is of a great marble tiger. The tiger stirs, rises to its feet, then rears as if to spring. I turn to run in the opposite direction, toward Caesar, but my feet are so heavy that I cannot lift them. Already I can sense the nearness of the beast, feel its hot breath upon my neck. A moment later there is the pressure of its fangs in the supraclavicular fossa on the left, and again in the nape. *And there is pain.* I look down to see my shadow bearing the burden of the huge cat on its back. At that instant I wake up. My heart is pounding; I am gasping; the bed is drenched with sweat; and on the left side of my neck there is pain, as if that area had been badly bruised. The pressure of my fingers intensifies the pain that I have brought back with me from that terrible amphitheater, a pain that has crossed from dream to wakefulness. Slowly my pulse returns to normal, the pain dissipates, and I begin to regain a measure of equanimity. But only a measure, for I know that I shall have this dream again, that its pain and horror will be undiminished. Lying there in the ecstasy of having survived, I wonder, Had I died in the jaws of that tiger, died of a heart attack or sudden arrhythmia, died of fright, doubtless my next of kin would comfort themselves with the thought that I had died peacefully in my sleep. "He died the death of a righteous man," they would murmur to one another. Had I the breath for it, I would sit up in the coffin and shout, "No! No! It wasn't like that at all!"

Pain. The very word carries its own linguistic burden, coming down to us from the Latin *poena,* "punishment." It is the penalty for misdeeds; one is placed in a penitentiary and made to do penance. The pain of childbirth was inflicted upon Eve for her act of disobedience, and from her upon all those who follow. Immediately upon delivery of her young, a woman begins to distance herself from the pain that she experienced during childbirth. Such forgetfulness is nature's way of ensuring the continuation of the human race. It is interesting that Milton, reinventing the birth of Eve in *Paradise Lost,* has the masculine effrontery to anesthetize Adam during the rib resection. In book 8, Adam has just finished telling God of his loneliness, his sense of incompleteness. God has promised the solution. Here is Adam describing the birth of Eve:

Mine eyes he clos'd, but op'n left the Cell
Of Fancy, my internal sight; by which,
Abstract as in a trance, methought I saw,
Though sleeping, where I lay, and saw the shape
Still glorious before whom awake I stood;
Who stooping op'n'd my left side, and took

From thence a Rib, with cordial spirits warm,
And Life-blood streaming fresh; wide was the wound,
But suddenly with flesh fill'd up and heal'd
The Rib he form'd and fashion'd with his hands;
Under his forming hands a Creature grew,
Manlike, but different sex, so lovely fair.

Milton's act of anesthesia is evidence, if any further were needed, that a man cannot imagine, nor can he admit, the pain of giving birth. It is outside the precincts of his understanding. Had *Paradise Lost* been written by a woman, doubtless Adam would have felt each and every stab.

In the operating theater, both the patient and the surgeon must be anesthetized. The one to shield him from pain, the other to enable him to do his work without the emotional response that is natural to a sensitive man. When the surgeon cuts his patient, his own flesh must not bleed. Only the surgeon-writer lives an unanesthetized life. He sees everything and censors nothing. It is his calling to report these events back to the waiting world in the most compelling language he can find. Hours later, in the dead of night, he may think that the breasts of the young woman on the operating table were like the blue and white teacups on his grandmother's shelf or that the abdomen of the man presented for surgery looked shamefaced. But do not imagine that such imagery indicates a lessening of the surgeon's devotion to craft in favor of devotion to writing. It is, in fact, a sharpening of his powers. He is now most fully aware of his patient. Nor should he be criticized for making the literary most of what happens to him.

Many is the writer who has tried to make the reader *feel* pain in a fictional character, I among them, but all the pomp of language falls short in transmitting that private corporeal experience to the reader. As I have said, it is beyond the reach of words; it is subverbal. Just as well!

No, I'm not going to die. Not this week. Probably. Altho' it's only Monday. But really, I can't—despite that it would be convenient all around—because of the warbler migration. I spend four hours every morning in the park, scrambling up and down rocky paths looking for the little peckers. Alas, my once fine hand-eye coordination is gone, also my visual acuity, so that I see much, much less than I used to. It is disheartening, to say the least, but I try to keep my sense of humor. When the others crow about having seen the Blackburnean or Cerulean warbler, and I have not, it is a bitter pill to swallow—but there is always tomorrow. If my son were here I'd see *everything*. He is that full of filial devotion. "Look, here, Dad, see that oak tree? Now go up to the second fork, then off to the left and up about twenty feet, and there—a red-eyed vireo." When I have done precisely what he told me to do and still not seen it, he goes through it again. And again. Patiently, without the least hint of irritation. Everyone should have a son like that.

Take the three major branches of science: chemistry, physics, and biology. Each of these has created the gravest threat to the human race. Chemistry has polluted the planet and poisoned out of existence thousands of species of animal and plant life. Physics split the atom and introduced nuclear weapons, which one day will be used, no doubt about it. Now it's biology's turn to meddle. The biologists are busy mapping the human genome, and manipulating (engineering, they call it) our genes. They insist it is to prevent congenital diseases. Maybe so, but it will be used, mostly, to tailor the unborn children so that they will be "beautiful," or whatever the ideal of beauty is at any given time. They will all be big and strong and talented and *unbearable*. There will be no difference among them. All the infinite variety of mankind will have disappeared. As for plants, that is the gravest peril. Already there are but three remaining strains of rice grown in Asia. Soon there will be only one, as there is only a single strain of wheat in all of Europe. Should a new virus, fungus, or parasite come along and destroy these strains of rice and wheat, you may bid farewell to the future. Everyone will starve to death. Impelled by the greed of the corporations, the plant biologists have developed "terminator" seeds. These grow and fructify, but the seeds of *their* fruit are sterile. So every year the farmer must go and buy more *patented* terminator seeds so that there will be a crop.

You got that? There isn't going to be any future. This is all there is. So wipe that smile off your face and start trembling. It's all as good as over.

Okay. Now I can go back to my gewgaw-and-wisphood. Might as well. It's called whistling in the dark.

Dreamt last night of my mother—how charming, needy, vulnerable she was. Funny how a mother ends up *inside* of you—the opposite of how it began.

How slowly she dwindled in heaven . . .

Half a minute after getting out of the car in Encinada and heading for the nearest trinket, I discovered that Mexico, too, had come under the curse of Santa Ana. Which brings me to the nameless saloon into which I followed a white chicken to get out of the broil. The doorway to the saloon was curious in that it was incompletely divided by a plywood partition. One side of the partition was labeled *Entrada,* the other *Partida*—the separation having been made, I imagined, to avoid collision among the tequila-sodden. Inside, torpor: the metabolic rate of the premises had slowed to hibernation, yet I knew full well that it is just such a saloon that springs to sudden violence. Knives are drawn, blood spreads across the floor. I have read my Borges. A layer of sawdust had been cast upon the floor, through which half a dozen chickens high-stepped freely. Now and then one of them would lower its head and beak the sawdust. Along one wall were unoccupied tables. I took a seat at one of these. Running the length of the opposite wall was a bar decorated with blue and white tiles. In front of the bar, a row of high stools upon each of which a motionless man perched. Only the infusion of new smoke into the haze of apathy over the bar gave evidence that any of them breathed. I ordered a bottle of Bohemia beer and thanked Santa Ana for turning aside her wrath for a while. The Bohemia was cold. I was elated to be there.

A man slipped quietly from his stool, walked to a corner of the room, lowered himself to the floor, tilted his hat forward, and pulled sleep over himself like a blanket. Then all was still again.

Now it happened that one of the barstools, the one nearest the door-way marked *Partida*, was tilted at an extravagant angle such that its legs completely blocked the passageway. Perched on the very rim of this stool, with only the barest overhang of his buttocks resting on the edge of the seat, was an emaciated man, his head collapsed upon his forearms so that it seemed deflated. I could not tell whether it was the stool that supported the man, or the man who kept the stool from falling. The loose shirt of the sleeping Mexican was unbuttoned and hung outside his pants. From where I sat I could see that his chest did not expand symmetrically, but that the inflation of the left lung lagged behind the right. The tail of the shirt idled over a funnel-shaped scar on his back on the left side. Where an abscess had been drained—or an ancient knife wound? I thought about the fragility of the human body, how it can be slain by the single pass of a pick, how from the smallest puncture the whole of the blood can run. I ordered another Bohemia and continued to study the chest of the man between the curtains of his shirt. No knife so furious, I thought, but would relent at such a bared grief as this chest.

Standing in the center of the saloon, resting one boot on a shoeshine box, stood another man, squat and powerful. His shirt and pants uphol-stered his body tightly. He was slightly drunk, singing to himself from beneath a great awning of a hat. In contrast with the man at the bar, he exuded gracefulness and good health. I liked him immensely. An old man with a pale, exhausted look was shining his boots. Only his dry fleshless hands moved as he crouched in the sawdust. During this time I never saw the old man rise. Nor did he look up, but filled his vision with the fowl among whom he dwelt. At last the old man gave a final flick with his cloth and backed off. The big man delivered the remainder of his song aloud, emptied his glass, and tossed a coin to the old man. Here was a man whose appetites became him.

Now he was ready to leave. He approached the *Partida*, only to find it blocked by the stool of the sleeping man. It is always so, I thought. There is the cripple, the wounded, preventing passage. He awakens our folded, sleeping souls and harries us until we do not know which way to go. The big man paused. It did not occur to him to leave through the *Entrada*—or, of it did, he had decided to insist on his right of way. He threw one leg over, straddling the legs of the stool, then tried to bring his other leg across—but there was no room to do so. For a long moment he stood in his awkwardness, then he hopped and shifted his hips over the barricade until he stood on the other side. He made as if to leave the saloon, then suddenly turned and gazed at the back of the sleeping man. A look of cruelty crossed his handsome face. With a quick movement he raised one leg and kicked the stool out from under the sleeper, then spun and swaggered into the sunshine.

The unseated man did not fall, but remained clinging to the bar like an insect. His knees, locked in extension, did not buckle. It seemed a defiance of gravity. In a moment he would fall. He *must* fall. Just then, the old shoeshiner stood up and walked to *Partida*. I was surprised by his height. He was by far the tallest man in the saloon. I watched him pick up the fallen stool and, with infinite care, insert the edge of the seat beneath the buttocks of the man, shifting it slightly to get the steadiest set. The knees of the man at the bar flexed passively as his body accepted the gift of the stool.

The old man withdrew and lowered himself to the floor, where the chickens welcomed him back into their midst with clucks and flutters. The old man and I watched the chickens, he from the level of the floor, I from the height of my chair. Do we see the same things, I wondered? Do we have the same dreams? One of the birds bent to peck at the foot of another, where there was an open red sore. The wounded bird cackled and gave a clumsy flapping jump.

It was time to leave this bar. I did so through the *Entrada*, for in this saloon in Mexico I had learned how to avoid the loss of grace.

Three e-mails from the same loony, the severely manic-depressive M., who has identified me as her mentor. No, her deity. She refers to me as Braveheart. The small book she has written on her illness is dedicated "To Braveheart." I did edit it; she self-published it; and guess what—she is marketing it successfully. But I shall never be rid of M.—*never*. After two unannounced visits to New Haven, I forbid her ever to come here, so she wrote the other day: "Dear Braveheart. What if you are sick and dying? Can't I come to see you one last time—to say goodbye?" Answer: "Dear M. Yes, if I'm sick and dying you may come, but only after I have slipped into a coma." Meanwhile, she sends me ginseng tea by the crate to keep me healthy, and now she is going to her Chinatown to buy a music box for my grandson. How did I let this happen?

One of my loonies waits outside his home every night to be picked up by a UFO. Another has just phoned to give me the good news that he has raised his I.Q. to over 200. This he did "by spiritual means." Admit it: this is not your ordinary day-to-day wallow! Then there is M.—but let me, at long last, be a gentleman: she is managing, and on a level that neither you nor any of your kind would understand.

Reading Milton's *Paradise Lost*, book 7, I came upon that remarkable image of the "tawny lion" on the Sixth Day.

The grassy clods now calv'd; now half appear'd
The tawny lion, pawing to get free
His hinder parts, then springs as broke from bonds,
And rampant shakes his brinded mane.

I do love this description of the lion struggling to free his rump from the "fertile womb" of the earth. It brings back my days on the Obstetrical Service half a century ago.

Tomorrow I'm getting a haircut. I know that is nothing to most of the human race, but to me it is a Samsonian *occasion*. I have tried to impress upon Tony (my barber) the significance of his profession, but he is obtuse, more interested in his garden and his spaghetti sauce.

Last night I defied my metabolism—"Screw you, metabolism," I said—and stayed up till midnight for a performance of Molière's first play, *The Bungler*, at Long Wharf. It was mighty good. The Richard Wilbur translation is witty and delightful, the actors were superb. At intermission any number of men, I among them, could be seen slinking and sidling out to the parking lot to pee between cars. If you waited in line at one of the two urinals, the show would be over before you did it. I am told it is the first production of this play in North America. Could that be true? The end result will be that this letter is all the writing that gets done this day. I shall spend it deep in an armchair in L & B, a vast space at the Sterling with a herd of naugahyde *fauteuils*, all broken and unstuffed but perfect for sleeping off Molière. Sadly, I ponder the strength and stamina of Hercules, who crushed serpents with hands still pudgy with baby fat, while I, weighted down with years, am no match for a worm. Still, although I have said that old age gives back nothing, that is not entirely so. Yesterday I received word that I am to report for jury duty while I'm in Halifax. When I phoned the courthouse to ask for a postponement, I was told I could be taken off the rolls entirely because I am over seventy. Now that's something: old age has freed me from judging my peers.

⁊

Not long ago I attended the memorial service for a twenty-one-year-old Yale senior. Six weeks earlier he had disappeared. Ever since we had been living in fear and hope. But then his body was found floating among the bulrushes of the Harlem River by a woman walking there. What was she doing by that stream contaminated with chemical waste and discarded tires and from which an entire rusted automobile emerges? Perhaps it had been the flash and slash, the ribaldry of gulls that drew her attention to that place? The cause of death was suicide. He had left a note. Yale's Battell Chapel was full of undergraduates, faculty, administration, and library workers. Brilliant, handsome, amiable, witty, and kind he was, with a low chuckle like water flowing over stones. Our friendship was conducted at the library where he worked for the past three years at the Circulation Desk. Most days we visited.

His anguish had not been visible to me.

Might there not have been an inkling, had I been made ready to receive it? A preternatural calmness of the features, a vacancy, the same stillness of a museum statue within its vitrine?

My great regret is that he didn't confide. I could have whisked him away and out of sight until he felt better.

Sitting in the chapel, I addressed the dead boy.

Did it have to be done?

Couldn't it have been postponed or dismissed?

For whose benefit was it?

Where is the reason in such an act?

There is no decorum in committing suicide, no dignity—behave yourself! I said aloud.

But even alive he would have been unreachable. To him it was all as mercilessly clear as the primitive sacrifice. It *wasn't* a gesture, an *I'll show you*. For him there was no other way. "I do not feel joy," he once said out of the blue to a friend. We were a bit startled, but then the next moment he laughed to show that it was a joke. Clearly it was not. And I know that no one but himself could have saved him.

The service was presented as a "celebration." We were urged to be grateful for the gift of his life, and we were to take comfort in the knowledge that he was experiencing the joys of Heaven. I didn't believe any of that. Doves cooing on the window ledge offer more consolation. Or the scent of incense. His death had made survivors of us. Survivors have the habit of placing blame. It is a comfort to do so, but not yet. We were too deep in the moist delirium of grief. All about us the vast, reverberant chapel echoed and vibrated. We heard the pounding of our own blood.

Throughout the minutes of silent prayer, a telephone competed from somewhere in the chapel. I tried not to listen, but heard each ring the way you hear a snatch of music you can't get rid of—it's what the Germans call an *ohrvurm:* an earworm. *Twenty times* it rang—I counted—and I had the wild thought that it was *he* phoning from anywhere but Heaven. I glanced in the direction of the sound, half intending to go and answer the phone. Then the hush of prayer ended and the phone fell silent too.

I imagined the boy coiled tightly inside his secretive mind, standing on a bridge over that polluted stream, the Harlem River, his pockets stuffed with rocks, smoking a last cigarette, sending the butt in a melancholy arc, then the waning life that writhed inside him as he took the "revolting bliss" into his throat and melted into the black, corrugated river that was to become his solution, the solution of him. Perhaps, I like to think, he had been dazzled into anesthesia by the light of a misshapen moon. Must I envision the hulk, weighted with stones, now swollen with gas, afloat and rolling a bit in semicircles, animated by the sluggish, cloacal current, bumping against tires, trash, the steely blades of reeds? It is merely a parcel afloat that no longer has anything in common with the boy but that is everything to me. That is the trouble with the imagination. It doesn't know when to leave off, but rollicks over into unbearable horror.

In my lap, the bones of my hands are visible. Can it be that these hands, which are only bones, performed surgery, labored to prolong life whether that was desirable or not? A knife would have been kinder, more fitting somehow. To open his throat, then thrust a finger into the wound to make it larger, the blood leaping over my hand and down my arm. But no, never. Instead, I would hold his head quietly between my hands and look into it the way children look at things forbidden. I would not be intimidated by the mysteries of the brain: the gyri and sulci, the pons and the medulla oblongata. I would gaze and gaze until I could see the black creature that crouched at the bottom of his skull. I would reach in and . . . *pounce!* Grab it just behind the neck—I know the art of extirpation—and wrest it free.

I have grown so old that I am young again, unburdened with wisdom, and with a head full of bloody fantasies.

Let others celebrate his life. I cannot transform an apocalypse into a platitude. Death is the most absorbing event of life. I have watched so many throats straining to go or to stay, you can't tell which. It is what comes of a preoccupation with the flesh. Surgery robs one of much that might have been consolatory.

At the memorial service, tears spurted from the eyes of the distraught father. "Where is my son? Who is he now?" I asked this of myself. The breath began to flutter in my chest. A knot of sorrow closed my throat. Stricken classmates bore witness. The burr of two hundred candles softened the taut features of the mourners. We sang "Amazing Grace." Just behind me a woman's voice put on feathers and rose to the stained glass. Tapes of music were played of Pearl Jam and Magenta, his favorites—and that was that. It is a tiny victory that he enjoyed smoking and did not live long enough to pay for it.

It is weeks now since he discharged his fractured life like effluent into the river, and still, in a telepathy between the drowned boy and myself, his face goes swiveling in my mind. I see his right hand raised, drawing over his head the shawl of water whose soft siffle might have been his last breath. I see him turning on his back as if to fasten upon the stars with eyes that were refracted for air, not water. I see the river dining on the bobbing flesh-wreck at whose flanks a froth of drool has gathered.

If in death he knows no peace, when will he?

I see the Harlem running like drainage from a sore.

This boy deserved a Nile or a Jordan.

It is the middle of October, almost ten months later. I lie awake in a bed that gleams with moonlight. I am submerged in it, as in a celestial river, like that sacred stream far away from human footsteps, in a clear meadow, under an open sky where, on the eve of battle, Jason the Argonaut reverently bathed his tender body. It is the Harlem, of course, only transformed by his presence in it, with all his unhappiness skimmed from the surface. I see no discarded tires nor any rusting contraptions in the deep, black pool. Elsewhere the river runs two inches deep over a bed of gleaming pebbles. Trout pass beneath the fallen leaves. Not far upstream there is a waterfall. Nothing grand, mind you, but a falls nevertheless with a long drop of six feet and two shorter *cascatelli*. There is a gentle purling.

Hastings, Nebraska, where all the college girls are sweet and sinless and the boys are hung with great aprons of beef. They are the children of farmers, and all of them work at two or three jobs in addition to school. They begin driving cars at the age of fourteen, as they have to drive themselves to high school miles away and there are no school buses and no one to bring them. The countryside is brown corduroy, flat and charmless, but the farmers' love for the land is passionate, mystical. They leave it only at death or starvation. One is nothing if not pious here. Everyone goes to church, either Catholic or Evangelical Free or any of several other Protestant denominations. I had thought myself the only sinner on the premises until I learned that the majority of legal work involves family abuse, divorce, abandonment, and custody. My own long martyrdom is positively holy by comparison. It was a two-and-a-half-hour ride from Omaha airport to Hastings with two female undergraduates—sweet, all right, and pretty enough, but I like to have died. At long last we arrived and I could crouch behind the door of my room at the Day's Comfort Inn. But not for long. Soon enough there arrived two more maidens to take me to dinner, after which, having been congenial through a trough of lasagna, I begged off on the grounds of exhaustion and did not attend the lecture on "Religion and Death" by a Presbyterian seminarian, nor did I go to the reception at the home of Mr. and Mrs. Somebody. No, I came back here and am writing in my diary. Tomorrow I make *five* appearances.

This is prime Christian right wing Bush territory. "The Lord" is in almost every sentence; e.g., "Where are you heading?" "Wherever the Lord takes me." It is quite possible that only some of the students masturbate. Poor Nebraska! On the other hand, next to them one feels silted up with vice and corruption. Theirs is a pale, cool, steady, angelic glow; mine, a hot, flickering tongue of flames. Among the courses offered are Public Speaking and Advanced Public Speaking. Here cheerleading is an honorable enterprise, though chapel is no longer compulsory. The news that I had appeared once at Focus on the Family has given me great stature. "Oh, Doctor Dobson!" they exclaim in reverence.

How to explain the cloud formations of Constable and Turner? After the eruption of Mount Tamboro in the East Indies in 1815, dust spread across the stratosphere so as to produce strange visual effects, *including cloud formations.*

Never regret a hopeless love. Even to lay your heart at the feet of indifference or disdain—it will be rewarded by the faint outline of your soul.

୨ଈ

It is the day before Thanksgiving, and the library is beautifully vacant, all the Yale folks having scattered. Like Ishmael at the end of *Moby-Dick*, I alone remain to tell the tale. The damned e-mail has multiplied like fungus on a damp well. I receive some eight to ten messages per day, although the ones from M. can scarcely count as messages. It is expostulatory psychiatry. She *needs* to write every day detailing what she ate, where, and with whom; when she goes to the gym; what her shrink said— everything. If I do not reply on the same day she suffers acute anxiety. Perhaps I am sick—or dead? She goes to the phone and begins to dial my number, then she remembers that I have forbidden her to call me *ever*. So nothing for it but to write her a brief message of reassurance. The correspondence is in French so fractured as to be virtually unintelligible. Another e-mail correspondent, a fine writer, entreats me to read his work, says that I am his only reader and that he can't write without that stimulus —so of course I read and I comment. This is the only branch of medicine I can practice any more. It is called Doormatology. In one hour, I'm to meet a medical student who *wants* to be a writer. It's really touching the way the medical students seek me out here at the library. If I'm napping they stand around like cows waiting to be milked.

At Thanksgiving dinner, with a dozen turkey-shaped people seated around the table, I had a momentary impulse to stick my fork in a neighbor's breast and carve a slice. It is what comes of spending one's time in solitude. The more reclusive I've grown, the wilder, the more fierce. Who knows when and where it will burst forth? I can only hope that I give a warning howl before lunging.

2001

MIDNIGHT, NOON—THE TWIN hinges of the day, when the hands of all the clocks in the world are raised, either to strike or in supplication.

Translated from Latin the death of Petronius. Having gained Nero's wrath for his satirical writings on the empire, Petronius prepared to die. In the company of friends, he opened the veins in his wrists, then bound them up tightly again, thus showing his power over death. He and his friends dined and chatted and drank until it was time for Petronius to unbind his wrists again, whereupon he bled to death, but not before he had smashed the one thing he knew that Nero coveted—a vase of surpassing beauty. It is in the writings of Petronius that Nero's lovers, male and female, come down to us by name.

Strange how these hours of *keeping* have made me feel better. Not physically, but in the manner of the god of Hard Work when he appears before the dissatisfied idle.

Feeling that something negative is about to happen. Must ship some cartons to the Archive.

I have resumed walking to the library in the mornings. It is a brisk twenty minutes along Hillhouse Avenue, called "the most beautiful street in America" by Charles Dickens. It is lined with great oaks (used to be elms before the Dutch elm disease). The buildings are huge and of numerous architectural styles. There are many squirrels scampering underfoot. This morning a loud cawing: an entire murder of crows. I looked up to see a silver hawk being mobbed. Once I heard a still-living squirrel chattering overhead in the talons of a red-tail hawk. That and the conversing of the raccoons at three in the morning are my only hold on nature.

I have always considered myself ugly. And I am—ugly enough. Still, with doctoring in the library, the Ministry of Loonies, the daily e-mail to M., and a number of other submissive, not to say masochistic acts, I have grown one wing. Useless, it flaps wildly behind me. What strikes me is how imprisoned we all are. Whatever wit, modesty, and politeness are mine, they serve only to distance me from others.

Asked by M. if I fear death. No, I don't. He who doesn't desire anything can let it all go. My hopes of being a little old bald tubby man with money enough to eat oysters every day are shot. There is all this pewter-colored hair that sits like a cap on my skull, and I cannot afford oysters. Eyesight fading, I'm as nearsighted as a sturgeon fumbling along the bottom with its whiskers.

Remembrance of a long-ago happiness is better than the event itself— whatever bitterness has leaked out. But I have heard no laughter in years. Certainly none of my own. Now my dream is to have nothing whatever to do and make love to a fat girl.

I've been looking at photos of the Isenheim Crucifixion—the festering wounds, gray lumps, splayed and distorted fingers, broken feet. Thornspeckled, purulent eruptions. The Antonite monks, in their directions to the artist, stipulated that these lesions be shown. The altarpiece was meant for the Isenheim Hospital, which treated diseases of the skin and blood as well as plague, epilepsy, ergotism. Contemplation of the wounds of Christ was the initial step in healing.

Yet another blizzard. We are bags of wool sticking up out of galoshes.

Dreamt of three Chekhov sons (of course he had none). In the dream I am attending a symposium on Chekhov. The three sons are also there. Everyone is neatly and respectably dressed except me: I'm in shirtsleeves, baggy pants—my usual getup. Everyone knows about the projected biography of me, which I announce is "an absurdity" and "pretentious." As I leave the amphitheater a woman I know is playing the piano onstage. She is dressed à la nineteenth century with a bonnet and much black. She smiles at me as I pass. It seems that I am a celebrity here. Am I looked upon as a descendant of the Master? I awoke in a sweat of shame.

Lunch at the Yale Book Store. Don Levy, publicity manager, showed me a copy of *The Exact Location of the Soul*. It's quite handsome—red and blue. On the way out I met Mary Curnen, a friend active in medical humanities. She bought the very first book I signed. At the Elizabethan Club I met Paolo Valesio, professor of Italian, newly come. He was born and has lived in Bologna, now permanently at Yale. He is a short, dumpy man of about sixty with the immense charm of the European intellectual, very affable. He is mainly interested in contemporary writers: Alessandro Baricco, Natalia Ginsburg, Giuseppe Ungaretti, Cesare Pavese, Eugenio Montale. He asked what my field was.

"Son io chirurgo."

He was dumbfounded.

"Chirurgo! Amazing!"

In Italy, it seems, surgeons are worshiped and feared.

"They do not discuss poetry," I said.

He raised his hands as if to ward off the very thought.

After two hours of typing " 'The Black Swan,' Revisited," the computer gave a skip, then asked me to say yes or no. Being naturally agreeable, I said yes and lost two hours of " 'The Black Swan.' " Quit for the morning in a state of discouragement. Walked quickly from the library to the Medical School, keeping my gaze on the pavement at my feet. This out of frustration at being stopped and blandished or importuned by a dozen people in the space of six blocks. Avoiding eye contact, it's called. Pretty women use it to deny men access to their society. It works! I recommend this method of avoiding bores. I was not greeted once for the whole trek. Which threw me into a slough of despond. At the gym I met a sixty-year-old bachelor, a closeted gay, a deeply unhappy and lonely man who affects hearty Yalish bonhomie. It is both affecting and obnoxious. He needs to tot up his multifarious interests, activities, friends, over and over. It may fool the imperceptive.

I see that I am seventy-two and a half years old. It is too old to go pole vaulting from podium to podium, but I cannot stay here and find tranquillity, so off I must go. I hope I'll be accepted by one or the other of the Italian institutes to which I have applied. If I'm not, I'll have to go up to Troy and spend a month or two just to sit outdoors, read, write, and listen to many-belfry'd Troy.

I have come to the conclusion that the trick to escaping despair and horror is to keep busy, even at the most inane and stupid activity, and to invest what you're doing with a sense of importance and immerse yourself in it—no matter how ridiculous the project.

Meanwhile, the pilgrims keep coming. Here is a psychologist and his daughter who raises llamas and wants to write about those "tender, adorable animals" (I wanted to ask what their feces looked like, but refrained). Then an aspiring doctor-writer whose copy of *Mortal Lessons* he claims I signed when he was in high school. It is my essential and deeply rooted nerdity that causes me to let them come. Probably it is also an excuse for not writing and a way of getting through the day under the delusion that I am doing good. Out of sheer petulance, I accepted a speaking engagement in San Diego: *one thousand foot-and-ankle doctors!* Perhaps they will stamp instead of applaud?

I careen from thinking "The Whistlers' Room" very fine to thinking it of no worth at all. In the original story by Paul Alverdes, the terminal kiss between the two young soldiers was on either cheek. I added the kiss on the lips, as I had set the stage for it earlier. I wanted all along for the story to be about the fellowship of the wound, but it occurred to me that the pure love between the two boys would add poignancy. I hope I haven't made a mistake in letting that take place. I don't *think* so. Until one of my readers mentioned it, I had no idea that there might be a homoerotic interpretation of the dilating rods that are used on the wounds in the whistlers' throats. That was certainly never in my mind, and I would be horrified if anyone did make that connection. And no, the love of Benjamin for Harry is *never* articulated. Remember that he is virginal and would have feared ignominious rejection. The kiss is an impulsive act of the moment, unpremeditated. They are not, as my reader says, "a pair of lovers who kiss at the end."

Attended Metropolitan Opera auditions here. Most enjoyable. Did not visit Maynard Mack today. It is not easy to face a man whose existence is limited to so narrow a strip—without food (he cannot swallow), without drink, without sex, without mobility, without hope. The odd thing is that he has not lost the desire to live. It has nothing to do with faith in God. His Christianity is regular, studious, and cool, not the kind that grants you peace. I reproach myself for not visiting him. I envy the narcissist who lives in perfect harmony with himself.

"You," said the student at the Circulation Desk, "are Dr. Selzer."

I admitted it.

"My father told me that you invented the word *aqualune*. Is it true?"

"One of my lesser works."

The students are unusually *rambumptious* today. Every library should be staffed by a team of silencers.

Everyone eats out every night in Silicon Valley. The cars are all Cadillacs, Lexuses, BMWs. So what? There's no place to park them. The men are identically dressed in black, head to toe. Why? And why would anyone choose to live here where everything is overpriced? This is not my country. The Anthony Powell I've been reading, *Dance,* is the worst book imaginable. I have also Barry Lopez's *Light Action in the Caribbean.* Not good, but readable. Like Oscar Wilde, I shall have to write in my diary in order to have something sensational to read. At 3:30 A.M. I went for a walk in the dark. The leaves are huge, shiny—magnolia and citrus; the air cool and damp with an odor of sewage, only sweet: the odor of decay. Camellias blooming and dying on the same tree! The ferocity of the vegetation—bristling, stiff, knifish, and mustachioed. Lacking in decorum and delicacy, interesting but unlovable. One prunes at Stanford only to clear a path. The health of the plant is not at stake. It is a different view of gardening from our New England way.

The visit stretches out like an endless prairie. I am that most difficult species of guest who makes no demands or requests. Met a professor of medicine, the sort who cannot wait to disengage his hand from yours. It is held out with obvious reluctance and retracted after a second of contact. Charitably, this could be shyness, but it is closer to aversion, possibly stemming from a fear of contagion or intimacy. Such quick manual recoil makes of the simplest act of congeniality, a handshake, a dark venture into the perverse. The hand so rejected cannot help but feel insulted.

Walked to the center of campus. Extraordinary display of plant and bird life, mostly unknown to me. Everything is precisely situated. There is a splendor about it, though practiced, not spontaneous. Tall, dense hedges reach up to touch the eaves of the roofs, hiding the houses, giving them a bashful, furtive look. One imagines the most outré behavior behind and beneath. At noon it is practically deserted. A total absence of insectivora. Chatted with a young man from Rochester, an environmental engineer who will start business school in the fall.

HE: You are a fascinating man. I felt an immediate attraction to you.
ME: We're both New Englanders, can smell it on each other.
HE: What's your name? I want to read one of your books.
ME: *(Thought but not spoken.)* Will you come and live with me?

Suddenly whatever had gone wrong with the visit was set to rights with the appearance of a robin-sized bird, with deep blue crown and back, dark eyeliner, and pale underparts. A shrieky, raspy song. *What is it?*

Sitting by the hotel pool dressed in jacket, vest, and sweater. People swimming. I feel quite isolated, far away. I think of Chekhov crossing

Siberia before there was a railroad, spitting blood. Why did he do it? To prove that he was not dying but young, vigorous, manly? On another level he was fleeing for his life, and from the tuberculosis, as from any sexual entanglements. It all sounds terribly familiar to me.

It is ten years since my last cigarette, a thought that gives me neither pride nor satisfaction. Ten years ago I was not flesh and blood but something made of ink and smoke. What to some is a noxious miasma, to others is a perfumed cloud. The greatest insult to my writing was not the coma of Legionnaires' disease but the deprivation of tobacco. How the imagination thrived in the milieu of smoke! Wrenched out of that congenial atmosphere, it has accumulated barnacles and rusted like a sunken vessel.

I can no longer see the numbers on the crossword puzzle. The cataracts are ripening. Until this year, I may have been something of a writer; now I do but make sport with words. Hair, teeth, eyesight, taste, everything fades with advancing age. Only lust lives on and even flourishes in the elderly. I see it in the starved glances of my cronies when a pretty woman walks by. I'm chock-full of it myself. I wrote to my Finnish friend Hilkka and gave her a thousand kisses; but with kissing, as with literary reputation, word of mouth is best. The truth is that I love Hilkka only when I am writing to her. The very act of writing a letter causes the rebirth of love, but the feeling leaves me the moment I sign my name. It is the mark of an insincere man, an actor. My letters to her are performances in which it is no longer Hilkka and Dick, it is "Hilkka" and "Dick," their disembodied ideals.

Home from Troy only three days, and my nose is still full of the smells of childhood: damp wool, new linoleum, mothballs, candlewax, horse manure, pickled herring, freshly slaughtered chicken, carbolic acid, tincture of merthiolate, wet plaster of Paris, gangrene. It is a city made of wood, brick, and stone, inhabited by its living and its dead, for there is more than a touch of the necropolis about Troy, the way the mausolea of Oakwood Cemetery are repeated in the nineteenth-century buildings of every style. You can walk for blocks without sighting a living Trojan, then your gaze is attracted by a movement on the periphery of vision. One of your *muscae volitantes?* No, it is a woman of a certain age leaning from a third-story balcony. She is smoking a languid cigarette and wears a bathrobe of thick soft cotton with a raised pattern exactly like the bed-spreads of eld. Her hair, enhaloed by smoke, is wavy and indistinct. We watch each other in silence, or rather in wordless confrontation.

Fifth Avenue between Jacob and Federal Streets is an anthracite-colored slum. My house is vacant, boarded up, the victim of a house fire. Here and there a heap of rubble, a garbage-strewn vacant lot, a decrepit windowless tenement. But these, too, are part of the city, along with its Tiffany windows, marble mansions, and elaborate ironwork. Could this cindery, moribund town be where the Industrial Revolution reached its zenith in the Northeast?

Nature was in a capricious mood when she saw to it that I was born and raised in Troy. I was unlike any of my tribesfellows, many of whom, it must be said, were handsome ruffians. It does not keep me from taking up the cudgel in defense of my town and all who dwell in it.

Laurence Rockefeller has put up the money for Bill Moyers to do a documentary on the Hudson River Valley. They came here to meet me and the result was a two-day excursion to Troy, during which I was filmed everywhere: climbing the tower of the Crematorium, walking in Wash-ington Park, at the river's bank, on the stage of the Troy Music Hall, et cetera. Two full days of filming left me exhausted and a bit depressed. I was not paid, but everyone else was. Handsomely, I was told. The cam-eraman is said to be the best in the business, also the sound man and the lighting guy. It was an entourage that followed me around Troy. But I loved the whole crew. The low point was when I had to sing two of my mother's songs at the Music Hall—very poor! Now the producers will ponder and decide what parts they will use. Not much, I bet. There is, after all, West Point, the Hudson River School of painting, the Erie Canal, and so much more. I can't imagine why they think I can add to it. I was supposed to stay another night and go to a Saint Patrick's Day party, but I fled the town early Saturday morning. It was the first time ever that I was glad to leave Troy.

Already the events in Troy have slipped out of focus. A certain Richard Selzer went to Troy to impersonate another Richard Selzer, whom no one alive can remember having seen or spoken with. The imposturage cannot be refuted. Only I know how false it is. Again and again I ask myself why I did it. Is it to boost my beloved homeland? To bring the tattered old town into view? Perhaps it is just the chance to play the ham, which only the pathologically bashful are able to renounce. I acted the trouper, never questioning or objecting, always willing to be "taken" and "retaken." I will never do it or anything like it again. It is closest to vaudevillian pornography.

Lavish praise from the Boys Friendly, who are all reading *The Exact Location of the Soul*. Vanity and Modesty are grappling for my soul. Vanity is winning. But in almost every instance, my early vision of a piece, when the imagination flares up, is never fully realized in the finished work, which is always duller, tamer. Doubtless the reviewers will find this Achille's heel and strike.

I shed my religion the way a snake sheds its skin, with just that much ease, and never looked back. Not that life is pleasant or even satisfying in the absence of God, far from it. But there are moments in *human* life that are ecstatic. Such are the rare epiphanies one experiences when the essential *whatness* of a thing or a person shines forth. Such is the stone in "Fetishes," and the toenail in "Tillim." These objects take on a talismanic importance. The writer is charged with revelation, so that now and then his disbelief is shaken by a certain manifestation of the celestial. The other day I came upon an open garbage can wearing on its rim twenty sparrows in full flutter, such as to transform that low receptacle into the furniture of Heaven. In a moment it would rise and fly there.

In the last lines of Sonnet 94, William Shakespeare wrote, "For sweetest things turn sourest by their deeds / Lilies that fester smell far worse than weeds." Meaning, I suppose, that one who has been pure and is now corrupted is more base than one who has always been corrupt. Whatever the interpretation of that line, the fact is that European lilies are often attacked by a rapacious beetle, *Crioceris merdigere,* whose orange larvae can quickly devour a lily's leaves and buds. Since the beetle thrives on its own excreta, it makes a putrid mess of the plant in short order. Anyone who has been around a church a week after Easter can verify that.

The poem "Trees" by Joyce Kilmer is considered by the cognoscenti to be trivial and, at best, pretty. I think it has a silvery sheen and a lush imagery that is enchanting. That is why I can recite it from memory after seven decades. It has the expression of true feeling.

Read "Three Versions of Judas" and "Parable of Cervantes and Quixote" by Borges. Infinitely provocative. One enjoys the playfulness and the manipulation of lore. He delights in shocking the reader—making Judas, the betrayer, be God. His sacrifice was not over and done with in a single afternoon on a cross but is ongoing throughout eternity. He has sacrificed not his body but his soul. It makes sense that Jesus, who knew that Peter would deny him when the cock crowed, would also know that Judas would betray him. Judas serves God's purpose when he carries out the deed that was his destiny to commit.

Bleak mood not improved by reading Borges. The Princess Eboli in Verdi's *Don Carlo* had it wrong. It is not physical beauty that is the fatal gift, it's imagination. It turns every joy into bitterness. Its conjoined twin is vanity.

Made love all night long—in my dreams. Awoke with a kiss still on my lips.

Reading the letters and rereading the journal of Eugène Delacroix, a truly loveable man. I must look at a book of his paintings.

Good Friday. It is twelve days since a small bird, a thrush with brightly striped breast, flew into the glass pane in the well of Cross Campus Library just outside my carrel. Every day I have observed the little corpse, at first a full body whose wings, stirred by the breeze, gave a semblance of life. Soon they became matted and stiff. Flatter and flatter grew the bird, with dark seepage on the stone floor around it. In drenching rain and bright sunshine, the thrush has offered the remains of itself to my curious gaze. Only today I saw movement on the breast. A resurrection? No, a pair of flies crawling back and forth in the dirty work of cleaning up after fate.

Yet another Mortal Lesson: George Hunter, eminent professor of English emeritus and fellow Boy Friendly, is in despair. At age eighty his richly stocked mind is failing. He is fully aware of it and terrified. We are two of the six whose delightful privilege it is to open the vault at the Lizzie on Fridays. After many years of doing this, George has forgotten how to open it. Yesterday he came searching for me in a state bordering on hysteria. Would I come with him and help him open the vault? As gently as I could, I coached him through the combination and the moves. His gratitude was wrenching. Once inside the vault, I listened to him discourse with extraordinary brilliance on the life and times of the Elizabethan playwrights. He has every right to open the vault. It is I who am an impostor, knowing almost nothing about those times. From now on, when it is George's turn, I shall be at the Club to coach him through the opening. It is the least I can do for him and for the Club. With my own memory slipping, I will doubtless follow in George's footsteps—only I hope not to be in terror of it.

Easter Sunday. Christ is risen! At half past seven Jon and I were in the loveliest spot, a road alongside the Quinnipiac River near Sleeping Giant, the river swift-running with standing pools. Good forest of mixed deciduous and coniferous trees, the birding spectacular. I heard the deep bass thunk-thunk of the pileated woodpecker, and then there he was—no, two of them! Also bluebirds, yellow-rump warblers, flycatchers, nuthatch, kinglet, black duck, and so many others. We came home after two and a half hours in a state of ornithomania. I am glad to have lived to enjoy this morning with Jon. It would be okay to die now.

Yesterday afternoon, "tea" at a neighbor's house. The purpose: to meet her newly acquired son-in-law and greet her daughter. The visit was marred by the habit of the mother, who is eighty, hugely obese, and deaf—to say nothing of the deep neurosis that afflicts her—of lifting up her dress to mid-thigh. When I asked her not to do it, she lifted it even higher and grinned horribly. "Are you shocked?" she asked. The son-in-law and daughter were, I can tell you. For the rest of the hour Janet was busy pulling the dress back down.

After lunch today with the Boys Friendly, Fred Robinson insisted on lining us up outside Mory's for a picture. With Maynard gone, Louis ill, George and Gene going dotty, and the rest of us none too spruce, it might have served as a sketch for Théodore Géricault's *Raft of the "Medusa."*

To the Yale Art Gallery to see the portrait of the Dominican Inquisitor Fray Juan, called *Portrait of an Ecclesiastic*, by Juan de Valdés Leal, seventeenth-century Spanish baroque. I may choose it for the next gallery talk. It is the particular painting or statue that matters, never the artist I care about, nor am I interested in the artist's total oeuvre. While I was standing in front of the portrait, a woman I know came up to me. She had driven a stick through her right thenar eminence (the ball of her thumb) and now has a fluctuant mass begging for incision and drainage. I suggested that to her, but she is terrified of it.

Attended a lecture by Harold Bloom on the image of the hawk in the poetry of Robert Penn Warren. Harold was, of course, brilliant, and a Falstaffian figure at the lectern. One of the many adjectives used by the introducer was *oceanic*. Somehow it precisely conveys the sense of the man.

Several rows in front of me, a woman in a red dress sat, or rather writhed. She was in constant motion—seething, swaying, wriggling, contorting her shoulders and neck, working the bones inside her skin as though she were being bitten or suffered some intense internal itch. It was the athetosis of some severe neurological disorder. Her husband's com-

forting and calmative arm around the back of her seat, stroking her with
his thumb and fingers—very touching. I, of course, spying. When they
rose to leave I noticed how thin she was and that the athetoid movements
had ceased.

Bloom and Warren were close friends for many years. Bloom believes
that Warren will assume the throne of American poetry side by side with
Wallace Stevens. Very possibly, I think. I surely learned from him today. I
met Robert Penn Warren once. The year was, I believe, 1954. I was a first-
year resident in surgery at Yale. Warren was admitted to the service of my
Chief, Gustaf Lindskog. The chief complaint was jaundice. It fell to me to
take the poet's history and perform a physical examination, both of which
he endured as patiently as possible. The diagnosis proved to be gallstones,
with one stone impacted in the common bile duct. Two days later I
assisted my Chief in the surgery to remove the gallbladder and disimpact
the stone from his bile duct. So I might tell Harold Bloom that I knew
Robert Penn Warren inside and out.

Two days ago, in the mail, a small miracle. Roger Armstrong, a retired
professor at Russell Sage College in Troy whom I'd met a decade ago
when I was awarded an honorary degree from that college, sent me a very
old, very faded photograph of 45 Second Street, the home of my childhood. There is the very four-story house with its square bay window.
The south wall is intimately applied to the north wall of 47 Second Street,
which sports an identical bay window. There is the brownstone stoop and
stairs with the gracefully curved wrought-iron railing, the double glass
doors arched at the top. Just south of 47 one sees a portion of the loggia,
with two arches of the limestone mansion at 49. In front of the house are
several trees, probably chestnut from the downward pointing leaves. Two
are quite young, their lacy foliage dappling the front of the house. Parked
in the street directly in front is a wagon, its two wheels huge and seeming
to be made of wood. A horse wearing blinders is harnessed to the wagon.

On the seat sits a human figure dressed in black, perhaps a woman. She or he is holding the reins. The horse's head is turned toward the viewer. The wagon behind the driver is empty. It does not seem to be a vehicle designed to transport people so much as goods and services. Possibly it was the cart of the ragman or the iceman or the sharpener, or any one of a number of men who plied their trades in the streets. If the person holding the reins is a woman, possibly it could have been used to bring someone to the doctor's office.

Roger Armstrong must be the kindest, most thoughtful of that superior tribe called Trojans. I love this photograph more than any other possession.

What was my horror some years ago to find, on a visit to Troy, that 45 Second Street had been destroyed by Philistines. A thousand years in Dante's Inferno to those who deconsecrated that holy site! The dignified red-brick facade was torn off and replaced by a fake white "brick" applied in the wrong direction. The bay window had been replaced by a deep raw slash across the upper face of the building that has all the charm of a machete wound. Only the high front stoop, with its brownstone stairs and the curved wrought-iron railing, remained to give evidence of the former glory. I should have preferred a ruin, a strew of stones among which tumble one might loiter in exquisite morbidity. Had I been present at the defacement, its perpetrators would have had to peel my flesh from the bricks.

Birding this morning in a desultory manner. Without my sons it becomes a bit languid. I guess I just don't care enough, keep no lists, am not avid. Plus I am not very happy these days, can't say why. Still, at age seventy-three to be able to birdwatch without pain is a blessing, and I did see my first yellow warbler of the season. Also a black-crowned night heron standing in the river not ten feet away. For the first time I could fully appreciate his thick, powerful beak. Female cowbird, rapacious creature. Pair of mergansers in breeding plumage. A swan in low, whistling flight.

Came across a poem by the Hungarian poet Jenõ Dsida that my friend Ferenc Gyorgyey, then director of the Yale Medical Historical Library, conned me into translating in 1981. This without my knowing a word of that impossible language. It was not really a translation so much as a free adaptation. Ferenc declared himself delighted. It took six months of sweaty effort. The poem was then promptly lost by me and by Ferenc. It took him three years to find it.

The letters of Gustave Flaubert reveal him to have been a deeply neurotic man, focused on his own moods and symptoms and overreacting, it seems to me. Upon the death of his beloved mother he wrote, "I am exhausted and grief-stricken." It is *the order of the symptoms* that impresses. In later years he is disgruntled, dyspeptic, fed up with everyone and everything. Aside from his mother, he really didn't like women. George Sand was the exception, and she was addressed as Chère Maître, in the masculine. Still, the letters brim with vitality and wit. I should have loved to know him. He was capable of strong friendships with men—Louis Bouilhet, Alfred le Poitevin, and Théophile Gautier. Bouilhet he termed his *accoucheur* (midwife), such was the degree of his editing during the writing of *Madame Bovary*.

Flaubert grew up in the residential wing of the hospital where his father worked as a doctor. He describes how he and his sister climbed a tree to peer down into the morgue where the cadavers were being dissected. I can relate to that. A childhood spent in the near vicinity of disease, death, blood, and gangrene is bound to affect a writer's sensibilities and predilections.

An hour of early-morning birding produced not much, performed without enthusiasm by me. The park is simply too full of us and not enough of them. One wonders if the park is not under a curse in which it has been rendered birdless.

Lunch with the Boys Friendly. Louis Martz has declined to a shocking degree. He claims to be short of breath on slight exertion, is exceedingly deaf, is seeing six doctors and undergoing numerous tests. He has lost a good deal of weight and looks sallow. But his mind is clear and he took part in an active discussion with the others. A pleasant, if worrisome, lunch.

Yesterday, a proposal of marriage from a woman in Indiana who claims to have fallen in love with me from reading *The Doctor Stories*. And I thought that *my* heart was flammable! Hers is of the driest tinder. I hastened to hose her down electronically lest she appear in these parts pawing the ground and salivating.

Thinking about the fear of dying that is all but unanimous in our culture. It was rendered acutely by John Milton in *Paradise Lost*. Adam, having just been expelled from Paradise, is being given a short introductory course in the world-at-large by the archangel Michael. Among other things, the angel gives Adam a pre-vision of one man delivering a fatal blow to another. Adam watches the slow death agony of the victim, and cries out to Michael:

But have I now seen Death? Is this the way
I must return to native dust? O sight
Of terror, foul and ugly to behold!
Horrid to think, how horrible to feel!

The impact upon Adam is all the greater when he learns that the two men are his own sons, one a shepherd, one a farmer. In the end, Michael consoles him with the reassurance of the continuing presence (albeit unseen) of God, and the possibility of reunion with God in Heaven.

Lunch with W.W. He showed me five of his newest poems. They are superb. When I told him so, he drew me into his arms and kissed me on the lips! This after a confession that for the past three weeks he has been in love with me. Coming from a perfectly straight husband and father of three, it touched my heart. I loved the lack of restraint, the unwillingness to rein in his feelings. After he'd left the library I returned to my carrel, where it had happened. A radiance lingered in the tiny cubicle. You could tell that a poet had been there. It is an event that is as pleasing to look back upon as it was to anticipate. It should have happened thirty years ago when I was forty-three, not now at seventy-three. I shall try to think of it as something that happened long ago when it should have.

Jon flies to France tomorrow for the weekend. His devotion to wife and children, his willingness to do whatever he can to ease their path, is admirable. It is a great thing for a father to be able to say that his son is a noble man in every respect. I have not met the human being who can match him for splendor and purity of character.

In the gospel of Mark 14, you will read that at the moment of the arrest of Jesus, there was a young boy dressed only in a "shirt" who had followed him to the Garden of Gethsemane. When the captains came to arrest Jesus, they also grabbed the boy by his shirt, but he wriggled out of it and ran away naked. That is all we know of this boy. He's never mentioned again. What I want to know is, was he on the way to be baptized, and so wearing this loose garment? Or was he a street hustler who had looked upon Jesus and thought of him as a score? Who else could he have been? I'm contemplating writing an exegesis or a story about this boy. Read Mark 14.

In "The Exact Location of the Soul" in *Mortal Lessons*, I had recounted an actual experience in which I hunted down, trapped, and drew forth in the jaws of a hemostat a monstrous creature that had made its lair in the upper arm of a man just returned from Guatemala. The "thing" was the size of a walnut, covered with black hooklets (*pedicellaria*, they are called), and had a writhing motion by which it extruded and retracted its proboscis, testing the air. Naturally I described both hunter and prey with all my writerly engine, implying that the beast that now swam in a safely corked jar of saline was Evil incarnate from which I had saved the world. Only at the end did I reveal that it was the larva of the botfly. Thousands of readers were repulsed and outraged and let me know they didn't believe a word of it. I was an arrant liar who would stoop to any depth to frighten or offend the public.

But then came Iowa City, where I had gone some twenty years later to give readings from my work. While resting between appearances, I thumbed an issue of the *Journal of the American Medical Association* and came upon an article on the treatment of *furuncular myiasis:* secondary invasion of the skin by the larva of the botfly. This invasion, wrote the author, is treated by laying strips of raw bacon over the swelling, a nodule-cum-aperture "as vividly described by Selzer, R. in *Mortal Lessons.*" You can imagine the eagerness with which I read that in three hours or so the larva will have moved sufficiently into the bacon so that it can be grasped with a forceps and extracted. It was described in the learned journal as "a moving form with white spiracles and distinctive black hooklets around the abdominal segments." Some dexterity, cautioned the author, is required to snare the larva as the bacon is slowly lifted, lest the creature retreat to subcutaneous safety. Colored photographs documented the case presented in the article. So! At last the world had learned yet another mortal lesson, and sweet vindication was mine.

The notion of the Boy in the Shirt is fascinating. Who *was* he, in his expensive fine linen shirt? Was it the gift of a homosexual client? Or was he, in fact, the one resurrected by Jesus? Did he want to warn Jesus of the treachery of Judas? I'm absolutely riveted by this bit of the Scriptures that has, at once, no meaning, and yet means everything.

Rummaging in the carrel, I came across a portion of my last Grand Rounds, delivered in the old Fitkin Amphitheatre of the Yale School of Medicine. It was the last Saturday of December, 1985. The audience consisted of my fellow surgeons, faculty, interns, residents, nurses, and students:

Last Grand Rounds
From now on I will not call myself Doctor, nor ever again wear a white coat. After a lifetime spent in the operating rooms and on the wards of this hospital, it is with a sensual greediness not unlike lust that I separate myself from the world of medicine. But what will I do now? Up to now I have struggled along the border between good and evil, with here and there an inconspicuous lapse to the other side. So far as I know, my only two crimes were to have been born in Troy, New York, and to have practiced surgery in New Haven, Connecticut. A surgeon doesn't get to commit but a fraction of the sins to which everyone else is entitled. So first thing I'll do is go out and break every one of the Ten Commandments.

Ah, the hot fits of youth! All those passions, long since flown away, will, like Noah's dove, come back to the ark to roost. I'm all for sin and vice, the prospect of everything caving in—a grand mess. Now I shall sip a choicer wine and make romantic overtures to women, saying things like *Who can know the year, my dear / When an old man's bones grow cold?* Or this: *What needst thou the black tents of thy people / When thou hast the red pavilion of my heart?* Show me the woman who could resist that, and I'll show you a woman whose heart is a potato.

Mostly I shall write. With what a childish pleasure I shall push a pencil about on a sheet of paper, crossing out words, rearranging the order of a sentence for no other reason than that I like the look of it on the page. Now and then there will perhaps be a small reminder of me—a book or an article, a story, either droll or melancholy. You will catch sight of it somewhere and remember that I too passed through these corridors. It is a pleasant notion that even as I grow older my books may remain young and able to travel to far-off places, winning for me friends from Bridgeport to Singapore, long after I shall have become too rheumatoid to go anywhere. In short, I shall pursue the mirage of Art. To do so I shall deal less in facts than in mysteries. I shall live in a state of eagerness, what John Keats, another writing doctor, called a state of *diligent indolence*. To me it seems a good way of being both bee and flower and of actively pollinating the world with words.

It has been said by one of you that I do not tell the truth about medicine in my writings. Congratulations to him who knows for certain what the truth is, and wherein it lies. I can only guess and surmise. Anyone who reads my books with the idea that he is going to improve his health or learn the ins and outs of surgery is sorely mistaken. All my reader can possibly come away with is a hint, a suggestion, an inkling of mortality.

How do I feel? Somewhere between contentment and longing— where all of us are, really. Contentment over a task completed with more or less credit, at least not in a state of flagrant disgrace; contentment, too, over the prospect of pleasure from the practice of new work, new experience, new friends. All the longing is for the loss—I feel it already—of the old life spent on the wards and in my hospital of thirty-one years. To depart from the workshop where one has labored all his life, and from the very labor for which one has trained all his life—work to which I was blooded at my father's knee—and from the patients, students, colleagues, nurses, orderlies, technicians, the whole host of those who labored in the same vineyard: it is not to be done with a cheery wave of the hand. What happens after January 1 depends on the faithfulness of that fickle companion, the Muse. Should she abandon me, there's no telling what will become of me. If some day it should happen that a drenched and bedraggled creature should drag itself to the front door of the Yale–New Haven Hospital, claiming to be the remnant of what was once long ago an assistant clinical professor of surgery at Yale, do not, I pray, sweep the saucer-eyed wretch into the alley but take him in, give him a bath, feed him oatmeal with a wooden spoon, then prop him up at an operating table and let him clamp a few more bleeders before he dies.

I had not read this since it was presented in 1985. It seems to me now a rough piece of work, unpolished, a bit clumsy, but heartfelt—and my heart was breaking. It took all my courage to speak these words. Even now, tears well up at the recollection.

The only news is that I am more grouchy than ever. My eccentricities are notorious in the city. But this happened today:

I was sitting on a shady bench near the library at 8:15 waiting for it to open at 8:30. A family of three approached: father, mother, and son aged around thirty. The father spoke.

"Do you mind if my wife shares your bench?"

"Of course not. Why don't the three of you sit here and I'll sit in the sunshine."

There followed moments of mutual protestation, then the father looked at me strangely and asked point-blank: "Are you Richard Selzer?"

Before I could dissemble, I had said that I was. How did he know? He had recognized me from the photo on one of my books, and he was hugely pleased with himself for having done so. It is a family from North Carolina. The man has read all of my books.

"You have a following."

"First I know of it."

Then I told him he had ruined the whole day, as my head was now so swollen that I couldn't write a word. With that I left them on the bench and went inside to the library. I was right. I haven't written a word all day. But I'm in correspondence with the curator of Prints and Manuscripts at the John Rylands Library in Manchester, England, about an illustration from Mark. He informs me that the "Boy" in the plate of the Agony in the Garden is not the "Boy" at all, but Judas Iscariot. He could be right, and that might be what the artist intended, but one look at this picture and you *know* it's the Boy. The eroticism in the involvement of the two is obvious. Anyway, I don't *care* what really happened that night in the Garden of Gethsemane. I'm going to make it up. It is the height of arrogance to rewrite the Gospel and I will surely be struck dead, but I'm going to do it anyway, writing it in the style of Mark, with a touch of Ecclesiastes and the Song of Solomon thrown in. Pray for me.

❦

Try as you may to separate medicine from money, you will fail. People have been paying doctors since at least the sixth century B.C. At that time, the medical school and clinic at Croton in Asia Minor were famous. I have seen an antique coin that was found there, a stater. It had been used to pay one of the doctors.

Guilt is an inherent part of the practice of medicine. There isn't an honest doctor who hasn't suffered from it. Painful as it is, perhaps there is some use for such anguish of the conscience. Perhaps it is a deterrent to carelessness and indifference.

The die is cast. Tomorrow I shall be seventy-three. What with the decision to stop driving a car and the unforgivable gaffe of forgetting to meet a friend as arranged, I am in a mood to surrender to my beshrivelment and slide all the way down. There might be a kind of miserable pleasure in it. This morning at nine o'clock I was in Grove Street Cemetery. I had brought myself there to learn the *ars moriendi*. No such thing took place. I remain unedified. I blame it on the constant roar of the Yale Power Plant placed disrespectfully across the street. The noise is as continuous as Niagara's and nowhere near as awe-inspiring. There was no pale loit'ring to be done in that place, no matter the urns and obelisks that would have it otherwise. Besides, I do not think of death as sad; on the contrary, it's the Mother of Beauty, as we have been told. The trick is to achieve it with dignity intact. Now there is a prize worth the palm: to go without uttering a peep.

I have begun writing "The Boy in the Shirt." I do not want it to be Dickissime, but rather on-the-Mark. My pen will be a difficult convert, I think. It has worshiped in the same baroque church for so long, to induce it to a plainer style may send it ablotting.

My seventy-third birthday. Resolved not to desire that which is not readily at hand, to resist the feeling that life has passed me by, and to be satisfied with what I have and what I have done. Reading Ecclesiastes bit by bit.

It's nothing short of amazing, the falling away of the mechanical dexterity I enjoyed as a surgeon. Where once my fingers were as facile as they were gracile, and each possessed of an instinctive sense of place and position, there are now ten thick knobs hanging from my palms. I'm the worst mechanic in the world, although I have recently heard of a professor of polite learning hereabouts who can't even manage to turn a key in the lock of his door. I'm not that bad yet.

I am reading in the diary. The entries are handwritten in lined notebooks and all but illegible, the pages covered with impatient scrawl, blots, cross-outs, arrows, and inserts. I do not remember having written most of it. There seems to be an emanation of desperate gaiety and exhaustion from these pages, and a vague foreboding on certain days, as though laboring to contain a shameful sorrow. All enthusiasm for the task having evaporated, I went for a walk, met a writer, and made the mistake of asking her what she was writing. God should have wired my jaws shut.

After a quarter of a century of peeling, the front of the house—the front only—is being painted. There is no money to paint the other three sides. From the street, if from no other vantage, we are once again respectable. Here where there is otherwise nothing new, ever, I can at least step into the garden and take a few deep earfuls of birdsong anytime I want. But Saint Ronan Terrace is thought to be one of the grandest streets in the city. Just giving my address offers an inflated idea of my *gentilhommerie,* when the fact is that we can only paint the front of the house!

A pristine morning, cool and sunny, after days of stifling heat and damp-ness. The earth touched by the hand of God, as they used to say in Troy. I walked briskly to the gym for an early-morning stretch on the mats. Envied the bicyclists skimming along. It is a major regret that I have not kept the knack of bike riding. I wouldn't dare now, for fear of falling and breaking a hip. Besides, however would I get the bicycle up Prospect Hill or, worse, Saint Ronan Terrace? I am told there are ten-speeds, bicycles on which one can run up an Alp with the lesser toes only, but I'll wait for the speed at which the bike becomes airborne.

Post-op cataract surgery. Did the marketing in anticipation of Jon for supper. Made cream of celery soup and froze two large jars of it. Read Maurice Blanchot, then prepared lunch: sautéed bean sprouts, baby bok choy, sesame oil, and soy sauce. Ate it over rice, telling Janet that the day I can read again I am retiring from the kitchen, but for the moment, she is to enjoy the respite.

No, I don't believe that the Boy in the Shirt was Mark himself, as someone suggested. He wasn't a clever enough writer to insert himself the way Hitchcock put himself into the movies, or the way a painter gives one of the lesser monks or soldiers his own puss. Mark was a clumsy writer who had none of those tricks up his sleeve. Why would he have cast himself as a boy anyway, one who slipped away from Jesus at the last moment? Nope. I don't buy that one. The piece is all on the computer now, and I will have to decide on the final format. It will have to be part fiction, part commentary—a mini-gospel with interpretive remarks.

Told Kevin Kerrane and Paul Wilkes about "The Boy in the Shirt." Both are devout Catholics, Wilkes a religion writer for the *New Yorker* et al. I said that I probably wouldn't publish it, as I don't wish to die of *rabbia papale*. Next morning I submitted to an interview by B.F.P. He too is a committed Catholic whose chief curiosity is of my long flirtation with that religion. I told him about "The Boy in the Shirt." I am interested to learn that Catholics don't read the Scriptures as closely or as often as Protestants. Most are quite minimally learned in that area. It is enough for them just to believe.

Neglected to write to M. yesterday, which sent her into a panic. She couldn't eat or sleep and went to her e-mail every half hour to see if I had written. I shudder to think what my death or disability would mean for her. Meanwhile I struggle to edit her absurdly bad novel. What I cannot bring myself to do is to tell her the truth, that it is worthless and that she has no talent. I have informed her that she has much work to do, and that several more drafts will be needed. Perhaps if I simply keep on giving her further assignments she will tire of it herself.

Finished writing "The Boy in the Shirt." Best thing I did was to reduce it from twenty-five to fifteen pages. The whole enterprise doesn't warrant a speck more. If my interpretation of him is considered by the experts to be naive or mistaken, so be it. I declare myself immune to superior enlightenment. It is the prerogative of the unbadged. The delving alone has given me the pleasure.

Took the bull by the horns and wrote M. to inform her that the "novel" is so bad that I cannot edit it. Having said that, I told her it would be all right to come to New Haven toward the end of September when I will go through it and tell her what's wrong. She is way too fragile, however, to receive the whole truth.

This morning, the second day of school in America, my grandson, young gent Danny, decided that he didn't want to go. There were tears. I presented him with another "grandpa shirt" to be worn as a nightie. It has a grizzly bear on the back and is worn to softness. In return I was given the tiniest smile in North America. At last he went off to school. *I'd* have let him stay home for another year or two.

Made a list of my preferences:

Landscape: rolling hills and valleys well forested and with many lakes, cattle grazing, cornfields, barns, and silos.

Climate: New England variegated.

Language: English, with an enrichment from French, Italian, Spanish, Persian, and Arabic.

Religion: Whatever, or none.

Sources of power: Wind, water, sun, and peat—no oil or gas.

Economic activity: Farming of all kinds, paper mills.

Means of transport: Horse-drawn vehicles, narrow gauge railroads, bicycles, barges, sailboats, tramp steamers—no cars or planes.

Architecture: Nineteenth-century English, American Colonial.

Furnishings: Simple, wood—no plastic. The latest equipment of kitchen and bathroom.

Source of public information: Gossip, carrier pigeon, learned and technical journals, radio—no TV.

Music: Opera, Italian: Verdi.

V. has decided to "take on" Philip Roth. "It's time someone took him on." E. has again "strained my head" and must lie in the darkness for some weeks. D. is visited at night by angels in the form of shooting stars. He is deep into his marijuana and vodka, a blend of giddiness and self-pity. All three have at least the advantage of being mad. Their view of what is around them is clear and definite. The rest of us are conscious of our self-delusion, and this is what disturbs us. It will be what remains after we have finished with our dreams and ambitions. My own life seems to have been a series of jerky, aimless zigzags, spermatozoic, instinctive, irrational, an inborn error of metabolism over which I have had no control, only redeemed by the gift of language. Still the patient setting down of words upon page after page is not enough. It most likely will evanesce into wispiness, then nothing. The sole avenue of escape is love, but I haven't the strength (or the will?) to roll away the stone from its entry. Never mind. I shall always believe that our own humanity depends upon the accuracy with which we are able to perceive the suffering around us, and to be witness to it.

No, I don't believe in a hereafter, nor would I want to. Why would any self-respecting god think a sly, furtive, sardonic sensualist like me worthy of preserving? I am content with the assurance that matter can neither be created nor destroyed. My atoms shall perdure in some form or other. As for the religion into which I was born—Judaism—it liveth not as a faith but has become an intellectual and social club. Protestantism is also a cold proposition in most cases. Only Catholicism remains as a faith, but one that is up to its neck in blood and perversion.

September 11. The horrible news about the terrorist attacks! Terrorism puts everything else in perspective. One's triumphs and losses seem all too petty. Contemptible, even.

The tomato crop is dwindling after weeks and weeks of zesty gorging. The sudden sadness of September catches you by the throat. How am I? Best not to ask. Am I comfortable? No. The spoiled tooth aches. The sharp edge abrades the base of my tongue. Am I happy? No. I love not, nor am I loved, save by Pirkka. More and more I am convinced that our not meeting again was a good idea. The threat of a lost illusion is too dire. Am I depressed? No, only I cannot find anything to write about. This last to be said aloud in the same whining voice used by Danny when he says, "I don't have anyone to play with." As for sitting on my duff, rather guilt producing, that. Where I come from, you don't get paid for what you don't do. Meanwhile, Greenville, North Carolina, looms. What I dread most is being looked at.

Yesterday at the gym, a youth, probably a freshman, paraded his gigantic cock up and down the locker room, in and out of the showers. If it was gaping he craved, he surely got it. When another man's penis would make four of your own, you simply have to take note. But what will happen to this boy who is in the grip of his compulsion? He will spend half his life on the qui vive for sex—in parks, bars, steambaths—looking and being looked at. He will not find love; he will know fear.

Chatted with F., who is obsessed with Christ and Catholicism, watches the Catholic TV channel exclusively, but has no intention of converting. Unlike me, she feels herself to be a Jew, despite all. When I told her that I did not believe in God she reproached me with utmost delicacy: "Then that is your loss." I thought about my own six months as a Catholic at age twelve. By then, Confession was easily achieved. I already had any number of sins at my disposal. My best friend Larry, a late bloomer, had to tell the priest that he had told a lie, thereby committing the very sin he confessed to. Before long I had given him some hands-on instruction in more substantial sins to which he took with rare enthusiasm. I believe the Father Confessor was scandalized to his satisfaction.

Aah! 4:30 and I am home in the sunroom, so-called more out of envy and wish-fulfillment than reality, with a vodka at my elbow. In half an hour I shan't care to say whether we should capture Osama or not, nor mind that the neighborhood curs are barking compulsively. How anyone can survive without likker is beyond me.

More and more I have the sense that where in other men there is a molten pulsatile core of feeling, there is in me a cold, empty, inert box. For instance, I feel not the least speck of nostalgia for my years at Union College. I was as happy and as miserable there as I have been anywhere else. Why don't I cling to the memory of it? Perhaps it has to do with all the changes there. Of course it is co-ed. That's to be expected. The students seem aggressively studious and "focused" on medicine, law, or Wall Street. It is more New York City than upstate. The old buildings are still there, some artfully restored, and new ones have been tastefully inserted among them to preserve the architectural flavor. I seem to have passed through this place in a state of enchantment—I remember so little of what happened, only my unrequited passion for my classmate Gerald Coonan and the poverty that required me to work in the dining hall by day, the library by night. The torment of love unreciprocated is immense. In time, though, mine faded, not to be recalled save in rare moments of daydreaming, and upon news of his imminent death. What did I study there? Embryology, *The Waste Land* of T. S. Eliot, French Romantic poetry, Freud, the New Testament. If there was drama, music, or sport I did not know of it.

For Albany Medical College, too, I have little sense of loyalty or affection. I strove mightily there to succeed. I needed a scholarship and saw to it that I got one. I was hilarious but not happy. Only when I experienced the patients did I feel gratification. They gave me permission to live. The Albany years were passed in an altered state of consciousness. I mooned about and struggled with my lifetime adversary—fatigue. There too I had to work, for two years in the library and then for two years as an "extern" in a hospital in the slums. My social life was spent with two or three classmates who also worked in that hospital. Each had already embarked on the romance that would lead to marriage.

On the way home at six-thirty, the evening already dark, a sudden torrential cloudburst; in minutes, the street was flooded, the gutters foaming. A tragic aqualune shivered in a pool of rainwater, broke apart, then came together, but only for a moment, unable to sustain its integrity against another bout of fragmentation. It is a thing made of moonlight and water, an aqualune: insubstantial, fragile, sent into magnificent disorder by the smallest disturbances of its component parts. It is I.

Later. M. is en route and there is no hiding place down here. Tomorrow afternoon I'll take her to a reading of T. S. Eliot's *The Cocktail Party* performed by the English faculty and directed by my lunch-buddy Murray Biggs. I've just read acts 1 and 2 of the play and really don't like it much, all that talk about love and happiness (the difficulty of achieving either). M. may be too crazy to sit through it anyway. I feel sorry for the poor woman, coming here after a ten-hour bus ride down from Canada to New York City.

Imagine a fifty-year-old Chinese woman with a shuffling gait (the smallest steps), a continuous trickle of mucous from her left nostril, a small face which grimaces now and then and from whose mouth a tongue protrudes and rolls, then is withdrawn. It is M. She has just departed after two days with me. She brought the second draft of her novel, an execrable, blatant, bathetic, pathetic, and sentimental charade of her own struggle to find herself while torn between the Chinese culture of Hong Kong and the Canadian culture in which she now resides. It's the story of a young Chinese female psychologist in training, her black lover from Kenya, and the rejection of the marriage by her old-fashioned parents. I have never read anything worse. She hasn't a drop of talent, only the grandiose idea that she is a writer. There is no grasp of grammar or syntax, only repetition ad nauseam of her "dilemma." The character, like M. herself, suffers from manic depression. In other words, she is telling her own story. Manfully, I edited (crossed out and rewrote) nine of the twenty-five chapters, then gave it up. She left with the suggestion to rewrite from scratch. In the meantime I had to hear again that she is in love with me, has never ceased to be since she was in my writing workshop at Yale. Would I come to live with her in Canada for a while, at her expense? I would be her "dependant." I told her no, but I have a friend who might take it on, providing the allowance was big enough. How about it?

All that having been said, I could not be brutal. Only a cat can walk on eggs without breaking them. So I squired her about to this and that. She left announcing that she had had the time of her life. She is generous, free of guile, honest—and absolutely crazy. I hope never to see her again. I'd sooner the gas pipes.

This morning, feeling overheated, I threw off the blanket and burst into a drenching sweat. In a moment the bed was sopping. Needed to have a bath. Got to the bathroom, felt faint, tried to get back to bed, fell to the floor. Managed to crawl to bed. Pulse irregular but strong. Feel fine now. What?

I simply must resume real writing. Keeping this diary is fit only for maniacs on a locked ward. All I do is shake a few words out of my inkwell onto a page and call it writing. There is no ripeness to what I jot. It is all hard and sour.

I agree with whoever said, "It's not that there is too little religion in the world; there's too much of it." This jihad will be the bloodiest of all, and it'll last a hundred years. If it's true that Iraq has chemical weapons . . . and germs . . . and all these fanatics elbowing each other to get into Paradise . . . I'm pessimistic. Maybe we've seen the best of it.

Oh, gosh—everything is falling apart. Walking home from the library this evening, I bent a few dozen times to pick up a red-orange-yellow-speckled leaf for the grandchildren to see, and thought, *Probably it's the last time I'll do that.* The mood of the country is elegiac, morbid. And then we see the extraordinary beauty of the face of bin Laden. Have you ever seen such eyes? Such an unearthly beauty? And in a man with a ruthless heart, a fanatic. It doesn't make any sense to me. My cronies here claim to be bored stiff by it all—the academic self-importance, don't you know. But I'm *NOT*. I'm hanging on every scrap of news.

Walked to the summit of East Rock this morning. Leaves falling all around me, consecrating. Met no one on the way up. The scampering of small packages of fur and paws. A hawk's shriek. Now and then, behind me, a footfall? I turn. It is only a leaf giving voice as it gusts. Lowered myself hand over hand into the well of solitude where everything is clarified.

Of all the birds, the rose-breasted grosbeak is my favorite, bearing its wound all through life. Once, years ago, I was helping Noble Proctor, the great ornithologist, band birds in East Rock Park. The night before, nets had been set up. When we arrived, a rose-breasted grosbeak was trapped in the mesh of the net. It seemed to have given up the struggle to free itself and just hung there upside down. Noble gently palmed the bird and unclenched its talons. He held it flat on its back between his hands, then blew apart the feathers to show me the body, unwounded after all.

Read in the book of Tao that a son is older than his father. So that is why Jon and Larry know more than I do. That is also why they can back the car down the driveway and I cannot.

The function of a psychiatrist is to ask, "What are you thinking?" or "Tell me your thoughts," as though anyone *could* do this. Thoughts are everywhere and all over at any given moment, crossing from present to past to future in a split second. Thoughts surface and sink from moment to moment. And there is a risk in rummaging in the imagination. One is apt to turn up a memory so traumatic that one could not bear to think of it for decades.

What had it been?

The more I rummaged, the more real it became . . .

It had taken place beneath a great weeping beech tree whose branches hung their leaves in a circle to the ground. It was the perfect bower for concealment. I was twelve years old. My beloved father had died some months before. It was under the weeping beech that I had accepted the warm, dry hand of a smiling man in a clerical collar. The hand reached under my shirt, paused at the nipples, then reached on and down. As if to register its dismay, a sudden wind lashed the skirts of the beech.

"Father . . ." I had managed. That terrible word. Minutes later the priest was gone and I saw myself clinging to the trunk of the tree, trembling with shame and guilt at what I had let happen, a secret I have kept all my life, telling no one. Now the old nail in my breast pricks me anew.

Article in the *New York Times* about the custom of eating dog meat in Korea. A photograph shows three men seated at a table in a restaurant before a steaming bowl of dog. I recollect seeing a living dog suspended between bamboo poles, being beaten in order to soften the flesh. I believe I described this scene in my Korean novel.

Despite reports to the contrary, I *have* experienced happiness during my lifetime. Once only last month. It occurred at the railroad station, where I had gone to catch a train to New York. One moment I was hurrying along with the other travelers to board the train, the next I had stepped out of the crowd and mounted the high wooden armchair of a shoeshine man who gave me a welcoming smile. From my new vantage I looked down at the people, tense with the fear of missing the train and running for the track. Now I turned my gaze down to the large powerful black fingers at work. First they ran a brush across a pot of polish, then applied it to my shoes. Next came the long brush with which he drove the polish deep into the leather. And finally the soft chamois cloth which he snapped back and forth until I could almost see his face in each of my shoes. That was happiness. For that time, my soul did not aspire to immortality; it was content to exhaust the limits of the possible, as Pindar thought wise.

Another moment of happiness took place in 1959. I was some months into my stint as Chief Resident in thoracic surgery. The Chief Surgeon was a dour, taciturn Swede. With his aluminum hair parted in the middle, his icy manner, and his impeccably clean and starched white coat, he was every inch the Chief of Surgery. It was explained by his wife that beneath the frigid and military manner lay a shy man. If that is so, the mask became the man. His reticence sealed up forever what may have lain underneath. He was a man who had withdrawn into himself and was playing his own game in silence and secrecy. One could not read his mind. His style of teaching surgery was *à la stocatta*, as in thrusting with a rapier. On the rare occasion that he smiled, perhaps twice during my residency, the smile waited just in front of his ears, like a wary mouse at its hole, before skittering across his face. That we were a mismatch became apparent within the first minutes of my residency. In his presence I blushed, stammered, committed one gaffe after another, as though I were determined to win the scorn that I knew lay just beneath that Scandinavian scowl. Only once was there what one might think of as a human exchange between us.

We were making Rounds together and had just boarded an elevator occupied by an exceedingly tall, exceedingly lean black man who got off at the next floor. After a moment, I murmured under my breath: "Watusi." After a pause, the Chief murmured: "Masai." That was the extent of it. Two words. But in those two words what a world of conversation had been uttered! Elation flooded through me that I had found the one word that would pierce the carapace inside which this surgeon lived his bitten-up life and call forth from him a response. It was as if we were making Rounds arm in arm, heart to heart; a devoted student and his revered mentor together in perfect pedagogy. But that was it—and never again. And he was right. Nothing further needed to be spoken. We had achieved a sublime entente that a single word more would have fractured.

Given that there is no record of a Sophie Selzer (or Seltzer) having come through Ellis Island ever, I wonder whether she was not an illegal immigrant or one who passed through another port of entry and later migrated to the Lower East Side. I do know that my father, Julius, was less than a year old, and that his siblings were quite a bit older—ten and seven, I believe. Since Sophie's husband had been drafted into the army of the tsar years earlier and never heard from again—a common fate—then the man who fathered Joe and Stella was not the same man who fathered Julius. I have long held the intuition, no more than a feeling in my tissues, that there is Russian muzhik, not exclusively Jewish, blood in my veins. My father bore no physical resemblance to his siblings. Nor was he like them in any way, he being charismatic, brilliant, and troubled, they perfectly sweet and uncomplicated folks. There is, of course, no telling what transpired. But I am left with the feeling of my Russianness.

Last night Jon, Regine, Em, and Danny came for dinner—a wonderfully congenial time. The children lit the Hanukkah candles and we each chose the one that would burn out first. I won! I consoled Danny and Emmy with Hanukkah *gelt*. Janet made superb potato latkes. I gave Regine my ancient monocular microscope, the one that I used in medical school that my father, too, used in medical school. It was made in Germany, as she was. She is delighted to have it. I was delighted to give it to her.

✈

Remembering my "Avalanche" talk in Galveston, when I was overtaken by the conviction that this was the second time, a sensation far stronger than an ordinary *déjà vécu*. No matter that it couldn't have happened quite like that, I am unable to lay the ghosts of other lives I have led. Again and again I hear myself saying words I seem to have said before, see myself standing where once I stood long ago. Could this be a *forme fruste* of epilepsy? Whatever the explanation, I felt that *I had given this talk before*.

✈

A young graduate student has sought me out at the library, word having reached him that I was the resident physician on those premises. I have seen him now a total of six times. He is handsome, six and a half feet tall, blond, with blue eyes and a snout chiseled by a descendant of Michelangelo. And depressed. If *he* is unhappy, what hope is there for *us*—the homely, the tainted, the stooped, and the sacculate? He has insomnia, he tells me. I can well believe it, as whenever I have gone to his room at the dormitory, night or day, he is lying in bed with his eyes wide open. That is the way he sleeps—like a hare, on the qui vive. I am using hypnosis to turn the key deftly in the oiled wards of sleep. I believe it is working.

All these loonies and near-loonies who haven't the stamina to keep their troubles to themselves! I haven't the fingers for picking them off me. I long for a companion who is *not* depressed, an *amicus ridens* whose presence would banish sorrow and who would laugh easily like a cupbearer to Bacchus. Self-conquest is the only triumph that matters. But then, I'm no great shakes either. I am getting smaller and smaller. Soon I will fit inside a shoebox size 7½ D.

We owe allegiance to two selves, one in the visible realm, the other in the invisible, which has to be brought into view or touch or audible range—made palpable. So we are ancipitous, two-headed. It is our fate. Just when you think you are all of this world, you get a glimpse of some other. The minute you let yourself fly into that empyrean, you forget the limitations of what is solid. I suppose this explains why I wrote "On Seeing Fray Juan." In any event, "Juan," "The Whistlers' Room," "Letter from Babylon," and "The Boy in the Shirt" are all departures for me. Who can say a word about their value? Only that whatever their worth, in none of them have I been afraid to be eloquent. To be bold at the risk of compromising one's past is the mark of an artist. Still, in each of these pieces the same Richard Selzer is recognizable immediately. Having long ago found my personal note, I cannot break away from it, nor would I wish to. The writer, like the actor, must yield to his passionate and often violent vision, and at the same time remain in complete control of himself. The two are mutually antagonistic. Still this knife-edge balance must be maintained.

M. is seething with passion. I have become the dream of a lifetime for her. As my discomfort increased, I obtained (from her) the e-mail address of her psychiatrist and wrote to him, asking for his help in extricating myself from this situation, but only if it did not injure her in any way. That was two weeks ago and he had not replied. Today I heard from her that he had indeed received my message but would open it only in her presence. This is precisely what I had sought to avoid. She would be devastated and doubtless become very sick again. I ordered M. to tell the psychiatrist to destroy the message without reading it. I demanded her promise that she do this. I threatened never to come to Toronto if she read or heard that message in his presence. She immediately obeyed and wrote the doctor as I directed. A terrifying morning. *Primum non nocere* was my motto for thirty-five years of doctoring, and I cannot betray it now. It is a fact I have learned: psychiatrists are among the least compassionate of physicians. They are cold-blooded and indifferent to the suffering of their patients. I truly believe they are bored by them. So, pinned and wriggling like J. Alfred Prufrock, I must continue to be adored by this poor crazed soul. It is a drama worthy of Molière's pen, or Swift's, but not mine. For my sins I must continue the charade. At least I have not injured her.

All energy having been sapped by this close call, I lapsed into inertia for the rest of the morning. At eleven-thirty I walked in the balmy weather to the hospital and bought vegetable lo mein from a stand. The proprietor-chef told me that he was going home to Vietnam next week and would be there for one month. Of his family, only he and his sister are here. I imagine him scrimping and saving every cent in order to go home. Doubtless he will give his family whatever money he has left. But the anticipation of home shone from his face. His exhilaration was contagious. I felt much better for having seen him.

On the way back from lunch, I dropped in at the Yale Art Gallery for another look at the *Hero and Leander* of Rubens. It is truly spectacular — the storm, the circle of waves within which the retrieval of Leander's corpse is taking place, the numerous nymphs, no two of their poses resembling each other, the gray-green color of the corpse in contrast to the tawny shade of the Nereids. Then just outside the frantic circle we see Hero taking her headlong plunge from the high rocks. Her eyes are open; she is gazing down at the body of Leander. She is diving headfirst, her skirt falling back to reveal her leg. The oceanic swirl is made all the more vivid by the inert gray corpse of Leander at the center of the painting. It is the sea, yes, but not a seascape such as we know the term from the paintings of Turner and Bonington. It is a nightmare of the sea, wild and terrifying, that awakens our own deep-seated fear of drowning. The sheer verve with which Rubens painted this — it is exhilarating.

Rubens went to Mass every morning. He even once presented a picture in order to gain indulgences. But his Catholicism was only skin deep. He was a pagan. It would take a Rabelais to describe the animal instincts here portrayed.

Here comes Hero headlong from her cliff tower and wearing a red anachronism of what looks like satin. Immediately, we forgive Rubens this sin against truth-in-costumery because of the power and gracefulness of his brush and the truth in his coloring. What in a lesser painter would be a flaw, in Rubens becomes praiseworthy.

It seems to me, sitting all day in the Yale library amidst students perspiring over their papers, cramming for exams and patently suffering, that education may do as much harm as good. Merely observing and reacting to the world would surely give more delight and, in my opinion, serve to inform and truly educate one. Particularly if it is done while young, when the power of the imagination is greatest.

I am half wax, half wine. After one glass of the latter, I melt like the former when heated. It is a sign of second childhood (lovely euphemism for the horrors of senility) that every excursion, every encounter makes me sad, as though I am going there or meeting someone for the last time. In such an elegiac mood I want nothing more than to browse in a good secondhand bookstore, preferably in a village in upstate New York or New England, one that carries old postcards and useless artifacts — an aspersorium, perhaps, that had once been used to sprinkle holy water upon the newly born and the newly dead. There, too, I might find old forgotten books with pictures such as delighted my childhood.

Louis Martz's funeral was held in a small stone church on the Guilford Green, the Christ Episcopal. It was filled to capacity by Yale faculty and administration, family, friends, and Louis's two small children, aged eight and five, who scampered throughout. I had driven out with Fred Robinson and Helen, his wife. Fred, who is deaf, needed to sit up front, so I found myself sitting in the second pew on the aisle. Throughout the service Louis in his coffin was within easy reach of my hand, just as he had been all these years at the lunch table at Mory's. Of the Boys Friendly, Gene, Murray, Fred, and I attended. The priest and the crucifer were in white. The crucifer was a very tall, slim old man with white hair, so much more fitting than the usual teenager with his acne. The church was decorated for Christmas with candles and pine boughs. A triptych of stained-glass windows above the altar showed Christ holding a cup of wine and a wafer, Saint Peter with his key, and, on the other side, Saint Paul. They seemed to me of good quality, but not, by any means, Tiffanian. The service was the usual rubbish—Louis is now among the other saints in Heaven, washed by the blood of the lamb and awaiting our arrival. Such a lot of poppycock. One of the hymns was music set to "The Call," a poem by George Herbert. The oldest son read "Death Be Not Proud," and numerous prayers were said. The two readings were from Isaiah and Revelation, both including the sentence *God wipes the tears from every eye*. I stood up and sat down as directed with the unfelt respect a heathen feels in a church where one's friend has worshiped. I did, however, share the emotions of the congregants, and I found the proceedings intensely interesting. After the service we went to the cemetery for the interment. The day was bright, very cold, and blustery. The coffin was very slowly lowered deep, deep into the ground, and then we strewed flowers into the grave. The finality of that.

I long ago stopped thanking God for anything good or positive. It was just a bad habit I picked up from living among the gullible. I also stopped blaming him for whatever evil befalls. On the contrary, he has my sympathy. Omnipotence must be a terrible burden. "Do as you please!" I cry aloft to Hera and Zeus alike as they argue over the outcome of the Trojan War. Were I to address the deity otherwise, it would take the form of the Buddhist prayer: *Make me worthy to dispel the misery of the world*. Of

all the beatitudes, my favorite is Pope's Ninth: *Blessed is the man who
expects nothing, for he shall never be disappointed.*

Back in New Haven, I walked to the hospital for a solitary and
unappetizing lunch. Felt sad. Then to the library, where I wrote to Claude
Rawson and George Hunter about the rites. Could not do any work.
Asked the computer assistant to help me erase some files. He said, "You
are Richard Selzer. I heard you speak twice to the pre-medical society."
We chatted for half an hour, after which my gloom had lifted. To the gym,
which was desolate, everyone having departed for Christmas.

Three more attempts to make collect phone calls by J.: at 1:00 A.M., 3:00
A.M., and 5:00 A.M. All, of course, rejected. He has been doing this now for
months. At 8:00, I had the phone company put a "blockade" on any
collect calls in the future. That will only partially solve the problem, but it
will help. The man is in dire, unimaginable straits, but I cannot let this go
on. He has no sense of time. Possibly he is in jail or in the psychiatric
ward. Once again, the stupidity of closing the insane asylums! A dumb act
of the politically correct and the miserly. There is no place for these
people. And here it is coming on winter!

S. is conversing with the angels; the fingers of his left hand are several
inches longer ever since he fell downstairs, and, of course, this is good for
his violin playing. And on and on. Every Christmas it is the same: the
loonies decompensate. So much for the birth of Christ.

It is a fact that again and again my tendency to befriend the disadvan-
taged and the mentally ill has become a nuisance. Think of M., who is
obsessed with me, and J., and the totally crazed S. and the others. I must
harden my heart. On every city block I am accosted by the importunate.
How to avoid them?

Regarding my illegitimacy once removed, ever since I discovered it I have had a craving for kasha, cabbage soup, and blini. To say nothing of vodka. Also, in a letter from Chekhov to his sister, he begs her to send his eyeglasses (pince-nez) as he cannot see to gamble in Nice. He is myopic and astigmatic, another bond between us. What with my newfound Russian blood, and my myopia and astigmatism, I am at last becoming a fit descendant of the Master.

∂•

Puzzling over what Edgar, in act 3, scene 6, of *King Lear,* meant by saying "Nero is an angler in the lake of darkness." Looked around and found that there was a lake, the Alcyonian Lake, down through which Dionysus descended to Hell in order to fetch Semele. This lake is bottomless. Nero once tried to sound it with weighted lines but could not. The implication of Edgar's line in the play is, I gather, of appalling terror and guilt. Nero was a matricide. I may have this all wrong. Must wait for the Boys Friendly to return, and ask.

∂•

I hate holidays. Everywhere I want to be is locked up. I could have had the entirety of Yale to myself this morning—and didn't want it. I finished e-mail and diary at 10:30, sat still till 11:00, then went home for lunch. I WENT HOME FOR LUNCH! Five words that speak volumes about my dislocation and sadness. *I have not gone home for lunch in forty-five years.* Ah, me. Then this afternoon Janet and I walked downtown, as if we were anybody but who we are, and now I'm having vodka and preparing myself for Christmas Eve dinner at her friends' house. A stranger would take me for normal. I can't have this!

∂•

Watched through streaming eyes a documentary on the life of Tony and Sally Amato, founders of the Amato Opera Company in New York. Although I never attended one of their productions, I knew very well the struggle and the triumph of that lovable couple, both now dead. Tony was the brother of Salvatore Amato, Jon's beloved oboe teacher. Sweeter men did not, do not, never will exist. One saw Tony frantically waiting for the arrival of the sacristan, who was caught in a traffic jam; Sally serving spaghetti and meatballs to the entire cast and crew; Tony serenading Sally with an Italian love song—all against a flow of operatic melody.

I've chosen the painting I want to focus on next, Rubens's *Hero and Leander*. It's both on *and* off the wall of the Yale Art Gallery. It's one of my favorite legends, and I'd like to wax irreverent about it. With that one, I shall have concluded the art talks—I shan't do any more. But that is disgraceful. I'm reading the journals of Delacroix. *He* didn't quit, he just carried on to the end. I *love* Delacroix—the man more than his paintings, but I love *them* too.

In Rubens the great mass of roiling water gives the painting movement, variety, and unity. The painting is pure energy realized upon a canvas. The viewer is caught up in the wild confusion. The eye doesn't know where to stop. Exhibiting both audacity and excess, the painting is the product of a surfeited brain. The sea here is almost a kind of drapery, and at the time when Rubens painted this picture a good deal of Holland was under water, so the subaqueous world came naturally to him. The child Rubens, in exile along with his imprisoned father, hears in his home and all around him the roar of tempest and wreck.

In the absence of color (Hero's gown excepted), there is the dead pallor of vapor and foam, a bluish-gray reflection from the surface of the waves. Such a turbidity! The corpse of Leander is already empty of blood, an inert thing, livid, greenish, mottled, clayey, but with the ghost of the handsome young athlete still clinging. He had been a well-fed youth. The flesh of Hero is satiny where it comes in contact with the dazzling luster of her dress. How very far it all is from the rich and mellow color of the Italians. His is the Flemish body—lymphatic, sanguine, voracious, fluid. Rubens endows his Nereids with spirit and an impulsive gesture, an abandoned and furious impetuosity. This picture evokes a universal commotion, a tempest of swollen and writhing flesh. The Nereids issue out of the waves, almost lost in their surroundings.

Much more than the Florentines and even more than the Venetians, Rubens sees the flesh as a changeable substance, in a constant state of renewal. There is nothing dry about these Naiads, and nothing at all temperate, and nothing otherworldly. The painting is all about water and flesh, reveling in muscular activity. But what are all those hefty, plump, turnip-colored Dutchwomen doing swimming in the Hellespont? No, their flesh is more the color of moldy Edam cheese. They are thickset, inelegant, with curious fleshy protuberances, their faces lacking in sculptural delicacy. Their very bodies are voracious, even carnivorous, as if they mean to eat Leander. Surely they are not vegetarians.

Rubens's is a northern sensibility: a single flash of light from the lightning bolt. The site of the drama may be the Dardanelles, but the sensibility is in Holland. Rubens must have been "Rubens" from birth, even before. This kind of genius cannot be learned; it comes in on one's DNA. The tragic death of Leander and the acute grief of Hero are palpable; they emanate from the painting and engulf the viewer, who cannot but feel sympathy for these two. It is the child in me that this painting speaks to. Like all myths and fairy tales, it requires a lack of sophistication to achieve the maximum effect. In this, it shows a kinship with Dante's Francesca da Rimini and her Paolo.

Rubens was the greatest efflorescence of the renaissance of Flemish art after the final breakaway from Spain. There is only one Rubens in Flanders, as there is only one Shakespeare in England. But he was part of a general resurgence of art, and was hardly the only great artist of his time.

I have begun to rein in the fantasies of M. It simply must be done, but done carefully and slowly. In today's message I told her that it was all right to dream, that not to dream is bad, but that not every dream comes true. I reminded her that I am married. This because her letters have become full of sexual longing. The refusal of her psychiatrist to help me cushion her fall is inexcusable. It is the true example of malpractice. I shall have to do it as best as I can. Even this much will bring forth a torrent of anxiety.

As expected, her reaction is extreme. I can only hope that she will not have a flare-up of her mental condition. I am not enjoying this one bit. I see that in my wish to amuse her, I have lived without benefit of discretion. It is a lifelong fault, this need to please, to amuse. Again and again it has gotten me in trouble. Up till now the only one injured has been myself. The fires of lunacy—this is far more than I bargained for. Hers is a wound I cannot cure, for I'm the one who unwittingly inflicted it.

L'affaire M. is proceeding as planned. She seems to be accepting the gentle let-down well. I did not press the point today, only praised her "fortitude."

Yesterday I ran into J. sitting on a bench in the sun at Cross Campus: filthy, dazed, and bloated, with his meager possessions in a bundle. He angrily reproached me for something I could not make out, as his speech is worse than ever due to the tachyphemia (cluttering). He shouted then that I should give him ten dollars. I refused and told him that I would not ever again give him money. I asked if he were taking his medication. He struck a noble pose and declaimed that he was the first cure of Bipolar Disease in the world. I demurred gently and suggested that he needed to see his doctor. A depressing encounter. I need to shed these loonies for the time being. They are sapping my energies.

The loonies have let up. J. is doubtless in a homeless shelter being fed and keeping warm. M. is now on an even keel. The crisis is over. She has accepted that we are not, never were, nor ever shall be lovers. So that is all to the good. But I must still correspond with her every day.

Thinking back some fifty years to my unexpressed love for Gerald Coonan all during the years of college. How every night I walked across the campus from my room to the house in whose attic Gerry lived in a room at the top of a narrow, steep staircase. How each time I was afraid that he would not be home but out somewhere, with Tanya, his girlfriend, perhaps. On such nights when the window of his room was dark, my jealousy and anguish were boundless. But when I saw from the street the light in the attic window, my joy was like Leander's when, struggling against the fierce current of the Hellespont, he caught sight of Hero's torch.

2004—2008

WALKED TO EAST ROCK PARK, where I spoke to the swans on the Mill River. It helped that they are mute. One can more readily disencumber oneself to the dumb, as to the deaf. I presented to these majesties the plot of my Henry Hudson story and asked for a revelation. Instead, I was rewarded with an ambiguous plunge of beaks below the surface, and the raising of one wing.

Went in the car with Janet to order my new eyeglasses. I am entirely dependent on her to get anywhere beyond walking distance. Also I am less and less aware of contemporary mores. She answers my inquiries with as much patience as she can muster.

Now and then, I dare to think that a few of my paragraphs will survive to amuse the medical students of 3006. The thought does me good. I'm pleased at the possibility of resting on a shelf in the bookcase of some as yet unborn doctor. Perhaps he will reach up and take me down while waiting for the next patient. I think of him flipping open the book at random and smiling at the antique quaintnesses on the page. The act of writing is more to be savored by me than ever now that I stand on the banks of the Styx with Charon poling into view.

Every day, it seems, there is news of a medical, as opposed to a surgical, cure for sickness. Just this morning it had to do with herniated lumbar disc with sciatica. A study has shown that three months after injury, the patients treated surgically and medically are equally comfortable. What is happening to surgery is what happened to the British Empire. It has been whittled down to a much smaller specialty of medical care.

Time was when the surgeon was a hero who came galloping in at the last minute to flail about at whatever tumors and infections afflicted the patient. But no more. He is more the man resigned to the knowledge of his own limitations. Still it seems harsh to deny pride to one who has mastered surgery, from the intern's announcement at lunch that he has performed his first appendectomy to the Chief of Surgery's Grand Rounds presentation of his series of a hundred successful operations for cancer of the esophagus. True, there is an element of braggadocio in both, along with the satisfaction of having done good for someone else. Such pride is entirely justifiable.

Both patient and surgeon must develop a realistic assessment of how much or how little can be done in each case. The patient does so while retaining hope of a cure, the surgeon while retaining the love of his craft. In both, the flame of passion must not be allowed to go out.

Reassured M. that I would continue writing to her. Necessary for her mental health. She is quite manic right now, but I don't want to precipitate a complete breakdown. It has happened twice before when I ceased the daily e-mail. I am shackled for life to this unfortunate woman.

Looked up at the sky, while walking to Yale this morning, and saw a perfect half moon. Feel it is a reminder that I haven't finished the Henry Hudson piece, and that I am to get back to it next week.

Old age need not be a time of idleness. In my seventy-eighth year I write as much as I did in my fortieth. I intend to study Greek so as to be able to read Homer in the original as well as to crack my skull against something hard. I do not wish for bodily strength or heft. It is more becoming to make full use of what one has. I have lived the life of a small man, fitting into spaces that wouldn't accommodate the burlier of the species. A small person can give the impression of being even smaller, almost vanishing, of drying up into a few twigs and feathers, then blowing away.

The one impairment most costly to the aged is loss of memory. I cannot remember names or faces, even those of friends I meet on the street. In writing my memoir, I invented a ghost city and called it Troy. "The rose cannot shut itself up and be a bud again." When I lamented the loss of memory to Janet, she took the opposite tack, as is her wont.

"Were I you," she opined in the subjunctive, "I should practice forgetting instead of remembering. The past is not a bone to be gnawed the way you do." Such is what passes for a quarrel at our house. Say what you will about quarreling, it is familiar, and therefore rather dear. Differences expressed are a mark of vitality in a household that might otherwise be as silent as a sofa. No, I would not like to be disfurnished of quarreling. With whom would I have the small resentments and misunderstandings that are the mortar of marriage?

At a ceremony dedicated to the opening of the new Bass Library at Yale, I have been invited to reminisce on what life was like in the now-defunct Cross Campus Library. Having used that library every day for twenty-two years, ever since my retirement from medicine, I could hardly say no. In the prime of my senility I sometimes harbor the fantasy that I was there first, and, like those tiny sea creatures that secrete a coral reef, I have secreted the library around me.

What have I done at Cross Campus all those years? Not much, physically. I sat still mostly, now and then lifting a pen and setting the point of it on a page. Nor have I thought at the library. Thinking is a conscious act. What I have done there was to imagine, which is an unconscious act, more akin to dreaming than to logical reasoning.

This is not to say that nothing happened to me at the library. There was the time when a lighting fixture in the ceiling fell on my head, knocking me out briefly. The concerned librarian insisted that I be taken to the Emergency Room, but I assured her that I felt fine and preferred to go home, where in no time at all, I had forgotten the incident. Six weeks later, someone from Yale's insurance company phoned to ask how I had been since the "accident."

"What accident?" I wanted to know.

"When the lighting fixture fell on your head."

All at once, I remembered that such a thing had happened. The wheels were set in motion to assess any injury. An X-ray revealed a small subarachnoid hematoma at the site of the impact. Ever since, I think of it as a ruby that I wear on my brain.

No matter how old I was when I arrived at Cross Campus every morning, the second I walked into the building I became a boy again, and stayed a boy until it was time to take the Yale shuttle bus for home and a glass or two of red wine.

Interviewed the other day by a young man, Duncan Crary, who lives in Troy. The interview is for radio. He had come here two weeks ago and done an interview but wrote in "desolation" that the disk had been irreparably damaged, and could he come again? What! Deny a fellow Trojan his chance? Never! And so he appeared Saturday morning at ten o'clock. He bade me read aloud three excerpts—two from *Mortal Lessons* and one from *Down from Troy*. I have to shamelessly announce here that all three pieces are strong and, in the annals of medical literature, unequaled. One is a portrait of my father and especially pertains to his brand of atheism, which I seem to have inherited all the way to masquerading as a Catholic priest to give a dying man his Last Rites. (The real priest could not be located, and the minutes were desperate.) It is not uncommon among writers to have been denied the gift of faith as part of the cost of having been given the path into their imagination and the language with which to portray it. In my own case, the other "cost" has been the absence of romantic love and prosperity. Has it been a fair trade? I cannot say.

The second piece was a commentary on the human brain, along with a touching account of a father's shocking realization that the tissue slipping from the skull of his daughter was her brain with "its cargo of thoughts." These pieces deserved a grander speaking voice than I had to give them. A deep baritone, "vibrating with virile passion," would have done them far more justice than my tremulous old-man's nasal tenor. But I must say that reading them again after so long an absence gave me a boost of confidence that I have sorely lacked in later years.

This morning Kim Martineau, a young journalist from the *Hartford Courant*, will come, also for the second time. (Her car had been broken into, and her laptop with the first interview stolen.) It is not quite an epidemic of technical disasters to which my acquiescence is the antidote. So I shall be flung in the face of two small audiences. Which brings to mind the small poem by Emily Dickinson:

How dreary to be Somebody!
How public, like a frog
To tell one's name the livelong June
To an admiring bog.

And this one too:

Success is counted sweetest
By those who ne'er succeed.
To comprehend a nectar
Requires sorest need.

She goes on to extend that need to a soldier lying wounded and dying on a Civil War battlefield. At the moment of death, into his forbidden ear the distant sounds of victory break agonized and clear.

Now that is great genius. I feel particularly close to Emily Dickinson, having spent the weekend rereading her poems between two and four in the morning. (Upon the recorded recommendation of Emily Dickinson in her journals, I am also reading in the diary and letters of George Eliot, one of E.D.'s idols. They are worlds beneath her own.)

In a fit of worthlessness, I wailed to Janet that I am merely taking up space on the planet, that I do no good for anyone, and live only to rummage in my own imagination. Now even that has frayed and wilted. As is her wont, she rose to dismiss my self-loathing.

"To how many is it given to have achieved one's life work and still be around to relish the rewards?" When I persisted, she got up and left me to continue the argument with myself, more or less as follows: I live in idyllic remoteness from both need and beneficence, and in a state of lovely solitude. My only good deed is to take pleasure in the good deeds of others.

The bleak news of the moment, in addition to the deplorable level of immorality to which government and organized religion have sunk, is that publishing as an "industry" has declined almost to extinction. *Harry Potter* aside, very little fiction of note is being published. Politics has become the "in" thing in books. I have little hope of ever seeing "Knife Song Korea" into print, despite that my editor has declared it a "masterpiece." While I do not agree with that encomium, I must say that it is not a bad little novel and is quite worthy of publication. The only justification for my continuing to write would be absolute faith in my own genius or dire poverty, neither of which I have. I cannot think why I am envied by so many others unless it be as Dickinson wrote. There is no reason for anyone to envy a rickety old has-been and stay-at-home as I am. In place of going abroad, I drop into a nearby gallery or museum to be transported elsewhere. Yesterday, I walked four blocks to the Yale Center for British

Art, where I visited again the ruins of Hadleigh Castle in the company of John Constable.

The funeral of former colleague Jim Kenney turned out to be a High Mass at Saint Mary's Catholic Church. Twenty or so white-robed priests at the altar. Interminable chanting, readings, and eulogies. For a man of small religious persuasion (if any at all), it was a martyrdom to endure. No easier to suffer than that other priestly predilection—sexual molestation. Doubtless I shall be struck dead for having written that. I have told Janet to refrain from any such "celebration" when my time cometh, but she is not to be trusted, and I believe would relish the role of the bereaved.

All in all I am still avoiding the notebook that contains the preliminary notes for "Mister Stitches." I do not feel energized in that direction, which doesn't free me from feelings of self-loathing at such flaccidity of will. Perhaps if I don tallith and tephillin and pray for improvement in my character? It's that damned funeral that made me write that.

For some years I have been leading workshops in creative writing for medical and nursing students, and for resident physicians in internal medicine, psychiatry, and surgery. This despite my feeling that, unlike medicine and surgery, creative writing cannot be taught. The secrets of art are best learned in secret. Still, a sensitive reader can make suggestions to the advantage of the novice. Just as often, the new writer will create an image that will affect the writer of long standing. Not long ago I attended a public reading of their work by a dozen of the resident physicians. One of them, Gustavo, a tall, lanky fellow with a Spanish accent, read a piece in which he remembered his father's departure for military service in the country of his origin. At the time of their separation, the author was some twelve years of age. As father and son embraced, perhaps for the last time, the boy noticed a single tear on his father's cheek. A moment later, that tear did what the father wanted it to do. It hid itself in his beard.

All at once, the years of my own life went by in reverse, and I too was a boy of twelve. My beloved father had just experienced his second coronary occlusion. He was forty-six years old. My brother and I were taken to Saint Mary's Hospital in Troy to visit him. After a long time, we were allowed to enter the room where he lay, pale and gasping inside an oxygen tent. He looked up to see us standing by his bed. All at once, he smiled broadly and raised one hand to wave. It was the most courageous wave of my life, a wave of reassurance. We were not to worry, it said; everything will be all right.

Not long afterward, there was Mother telling us, in that melodramatic way she had, that he had died.

"Our Daddy is no more," she said.

For me, the memoir written by Gustavo, with its intimacy and vulnerability, went straight to my heart. It could not have been rendered more eloquently.

Visited the Anatomy Laboratory, where the medical students were dissecting the muscles of the back. I could not resist tracing out with my fingers the translucent scapulae that rise like hillocks just below the shoulders. They are all that is left of our primordial wings, still retaining, each, the gleam of a bird in flight. From there, to the Reading Room of the Yale library, where I fell asleep and dreamed of that church in Troy where, from a certain pew, a single pane of stained glass depicting the Flight into Egypt goes *ping* each time the organ heaves its Great Amen. Is it any wonder that I place little trust in a mischievous science that takes its pleasure in undermining the supernatural? Fifty years later, each time I see a depiction of the Holy Family on the lam, it goes *ping* in my chest. Awoke to the sound of women's voices, their low, subdued laughter, their footsteps on the granite floor. At a table nearby, a blond young man, arms and legs in the lovely strew of sleep that has built a wall of self-containment around him. I turn aside to spare him the molestation of my stare. Should he wake up and see me, the embarrassment would be all mine.

Home, to see that the sick lilac I had pruned down to a single stick and brought indoors is popping out with new growth. And only yesterday it seemed irretrievably dead. Felt a rush of gratification, as when a moribund patient rallied.

It is nothing short of amazing—the falling away of the manual dexterity of which I had so much as a surgeon. Where once my fingers were each possessed of the instinct for position and placement, they are now ten thickened knobs hanging from my palms. I am the worst mechanic in the world. Nor do I have my former hand-eye coordination. This is especially inconvenient in birdwatching. Having seen a bird with my naked eye, I try to place it within reach of my fieldglasses, but that is not often successful, as I cannot find my vision with the fieldglasses. By the time I can, the bird has flown away.

Four months to the day of my eightieth, an age that like an abscess has been ripening all year, and is getting ready to burst. Well, let it! To begin a new decade is to be a child again. There is a horizon, a path not yet taken. Time to roam "with a hungry heart" like Tennyson's Ulysses.

It is no cinch to write your memoirs if you are the sort of person to whom nothing much has happened and who hasn't met anyone famous or important. (Luckily, I'm not the sort of memoirist burdened with a conscience that insists on telling the truth all the time.) In lieu of experiences, however, I have had lots of impressions, a few gushes of feeling, and some moments of exaltation. That will just have to do.

I spent the morning raising Father with my sighs. His sudden death just as I turned thirteen has made him into a creature of my invention. The man who appeared today was no more than five feet, six inches tall. He had a gray toothbrush moustache and aluminum hair, like mine. He had narrow, sloping shoulders, skinny arms, and broad hips.

"His hips are the biggest part of him," Mother was fond of saying. It was a remark guaranteed to offend any man who might have been within earshot.

Once, as a small child, I was taken to Montreal to see my maternal grandmother. Of her I have only the faint memory of a small woman wearing a *sheitl* (wig), bedroom slippers, and a white dress that Mother said was made of nainsook, whatever that was. From these two tiny recollections, I have reconstructed surprisingly accurate portraits. (I have since learned that nainsook is a form of thin cotton made in India.)

With my eightieth birthday looming, it is fair to say that I am an old man. It is only in the act of storytelling that I locate my vanished youth and become an undergraduate. No sooner have I set down the pen when my hand is once again that of an old man.

For so long have I bent over this story that I have become hunch-backed, like another Richard. Probably it is a good thing to take one's time, to work long and hard at a piece, but I have not that kind of toilsome nature.

In the role of resident physician at the Yale library, I am trying to be helpful. Yesterday I examined one of the maintenance men for inguinal pain. He does have a hernia, but the pain he is experiencing is more that of nerve compression than due to an easily reducible hernia.

Today I met with a young woman whose fourteen-year-old son has been treated with radiation for an iris melanoma. The tumor seems to be responding. Now the boy discovered a nodule in the ipsilateral neck. He is scheduled for biopsy. It is an ominous finding. The mother is distraught, of course. I have tried to reassure her that the good response to radiation of the iris lesion would suggest that if the neck nodule is metastatic, it too would respond well to irradiation.

The people of the library count on me to examine, discuss, and suggest. This last patient's story has demolished me. Having shed my armor, I am no longer able to withstand the slings and arrows of medical practice. In the words of Walt Whitman when he witnessed the wounds of the Civil War soldiers, "This bursts the petty bonds of Art." Still, I shall continue to listen and clarify and reassure. It is what a long-retired octogenarian doctor can do.

Read again the Twenty-third Psalm of David: "The Lord is my shepherd; I shall not want. He maketh me to lie down in green pastures; he leadeth me beside the still waters." If for no other reason than the utter beauty of those lines, I regret my atheism.

Three wonderful days of birdwatching with Doon and his eleven-year-old charming Ellie. She is so quick and bright and observant. Janet and I sat in grandparental adoration, called *kvelling* in the old days. As for the birdwatching, the others saw so as to identify the warblers, but with my failing vision, and slow hand-eye coordination, I missed most of the little peckers, and had to lie and pretend I saw them, so as not to disappoint the others who had made the trip from Virginia expressly for my pleasure. I did hear the Baltimore oriole—you couldn't miss it. And saw the indigo bunting and the rose-breasted grosbeak before my cervical spine refused to look up any more. Also it was cold and wet on the first day, my feet were two frogs, and no bathroom in sight. But managed to keep this *Iliad* of woes to myself.

Home at noon, ate my own beloved lentil soup, and lay moribund until three o'clock, when I baked a bread, filling the house with that smell of sincerity. While it was still warm, we slathered thick slices with butter and honey and gorged.

Next day, *grace à Dieu,* the sun came out.

Undated

MEMORIES OF TROY

EMMY'S RIGHT MIDDLE LOBE is still atelectatic, though she is asymptomatic after seven days of antibiotics. I fear that she will need bronchoscopy in a few days.

Awoke at 3 A.M. and felt the need to go up to Troy. Remembered that day of long ago when the flu epidemic had laid low all the teachers at School 5. The distraught principal appealed to the more literate parents to volunteer as subsitutes. To my profound mortification, Mother signed up to take my fourth-grade class. For "English" she presented a notion of word usage that was her very own and no one else's: "Trees and persons have limbs: tables and persons have legs. Legs are never so beautiful as limbs. *Leg* is an ugly word that is to be avoided except when it is used to mean the segment of a journey. *Limb* is to be cherished, if only because of the scarcity of words ending in a silent *b*, preceded by *m*.

"Oh there is *climb*," she said, "but after that, you have to rummage." The barrage of *thumb, dumb, numb, comb, crumb,* and *bomb* that shot around the fourth-grade classroom caused her to press her hands to her ears in dismay.

That was English. In Science, this: "The fig tree loves to grow next to a stone wall. It has marvelously prehensile roots, has the fig tree, that grapple and clamber on the stones until the whole wall collapses. That is why you see so many ruins and fig trees in the same painting. In France, they are called *figues des ruines*."

O my God! I thought. *I'll never come back to this class again.* But then she went up and down the aisles pinching those of us who looked sleepy until everyone was screaming with laughter. For the rest of the day, she posed us in tableaux vivantes of the poems of Longfellow—"The Wreck of the Hesperus," "Excelsior," and "Hiawatha." By the end of the day, the entire class lay at her feet. Except one.

❧

Jon and Doon engaged in serious talk about white-collar crime, things like securities fraud and money laundering. Becky dying of boredom.

"Who would want to launder money?" she asked, and yawned to show that she couldn't care less. But she perked up when I told her that her great-grandmother Selzer used to wash the dollar bills her great-grandpa was paid by the patients, wash them in warm soapy water, then hang them on a line to dry.

"So we wouldn't catch T.B. or syphilis, what with all the whores in Troy."

"Dad!" said Gretchen, and gave me a look.

"Whores? T.B.?" asked Becky. "What are whores?"

"Now see!" said Gretchen.

"Once she had the money hung up to dry in the back pantry, and one of the neighborhood bums swiped it." Now Gretchen herself began to take an interest. "It all ended up at the Central Tavern. I know because your great-grandmother sent me over there to see if any of the dollars were damp and especially clean."

"And were there any?"

"Oh, indeed there were, and three or four drunken bums, too."

"What did you do?"

"I told Mr. Sweeney (the bartender) to give me back the money, as my mother had just laundered it when the bums stole it."

"And did he give it back?"

"I should say he did not! They all just laughed fit to split their sides, but they laughed out of the other side of their mouths when Herself stormed over and filled the air with imprecations."

"Impre . . ?"

"Curses and threats. You can bet she came back home with a fistful of nice clean bucks, but then she had to wash them again."

Janet phoned, said, "Are you sitting down? The man wants nine thousand dollars to paint the house and fix the leaks in the roof." I searched all over my mouth for one of the oaths I keep on hand for a rainy day, found one, and used it. Then fell into a reflective mood over the descent unto worthlessness of the coin of the realm.

In 1935, fifteen cents a week was what you got for keeping the coal stove from going out during the night or for restarting it in the morning if it had. It also covered shoveling the walk in winter, raking leaves in fall, watering grass in summer, and weeding in spring. And all with a civil tongue in your head or no fifteen cents. Payday was Saturday night, and the money had to burn a hole in your pocket until Sunday noon, when the matinee double feature began at Proctor's Theater. In Troy that cost a dime. The remaining nickel bought a little white bag of hot cinnamon drops to suck while for the next four hours Jeanette MacDonald first took umbrage at, then yielded to, the laryngeal blandishments of Nelson Eddy.

It is a long time since those drunk-with-pleasure days, and much have I traveled in realms of gold, but never have I felt such thrill of opulence as when I sat in the balcony of Proctor's of a Sunday afternoon. In the past few years alone I have made my home at the Abbey of San Giorgio Maggiore in Venice, the Villa Serbelloni on Lake Como, and the mansion of Yaddo in Saratoga, New York, to say nothing of a few dozen caravanserais of the Hilton and Holiday Inn ilk, where each bathroom has its three individually wrapped little bars of soap. Not that I have become blasé about grandeur, not at all. I still like walking into a great hall, a well-appointed lobby, or a burnished refectory and making them my own. And there are times when a draperied couch has it all over a mere bed. But the Versailles of my heart is a cozy wooden cottage with a front *and* a back porch, a working chimbley wearing a feather of smoke at the top, and, all around, trees of a certain age for shade, birds, and the resident deities. Put a meadow of wildflowers out back of the fence and beyond that a creek for music. And there let me take whatever more of relishment is to be my portion. I don't need much: one deep easy chair, my share of vodka, a few cigarettes, a kosher salami, a tin of smoked oysters, a fresh, clean notebook, pencils to last, a volume of Shakespeare, and a cat. It is the only place I would ever dream of having a cat, and then it would be only as a hired domestic, subject to instant dismissal. The real use of a cat lies not in its appetite for mice but as a foot warmer in winter, a purpose for which it is ideally constructed.

From a vague corner of memory, this:

Two small boys in identical cotton shirts with stitching on the collar and short pants. Their father is a family doctor; his office is on the first floor of an old brownstone house. Their mother is a singer. She has a small but lovely soprano that sounds as if a white mouse were ringing a tiny silver bell. The heads of the two boys have been shaved for lice. They sit on the dark landing of the staircase midway between up- and downstairs hoping only not to be seen. The slim older boy has flung one arm about the shoulders of the pudgy younger boy, the one wearing glasses. They have the inconsolable look of the princes in the tower. From where they sit, they listen to the sounds that float up from their father's office—moans, weeping and the steady rumble of their father's voice.

"You're going to feel a sharp stick and then a burning. One quick poke . . . We're almost done . . . I do believe I got it all out." On the landing, the two boys tense to receive what they know is coming. The bigger boy screws up his face and shuts his eyes. He withdraws his arm from around his brother's shoulders and makes as if to cover his ears. Too late. The younger boy's face is serious, grave even. You cannot read any reaction on it. Only, perhaps, a glistening of the eyes. A scream splits the air and races up the staircase to strike them where they sit. The father speaks again.

"No, no, you mustn't holler like that! It wasn't so bad, after all, now was it?" The scream cascades down the chromatic scale, then by some alchemy of sound it is transmuted into their mother's voice—*do, ti, la, sol, fa, mi, re, do.*

All that suffering of long ago. What has become of it? Dissipated, I think, diluted and spread out over the world, still part of the pain of mankind, as though suffering, like matter, cannot be created or destroyed.

❧

I used to think the past was safer than the Present or the Future. It had already happened and could do no more damage. Now I know that it is the Past to which we are most vulnerable, the Past that is most apt to slay us. Periodically in the springtime, the Hudson River would overflow its banks and flood the lower streets of Troy. I have a clear vision of Father wearing his overcoat and fedora, sitting in a rowboat with his medical bag on the seat beside him. He was trying to row down to South Troy on a house call. From where I watched in a bay window on the second floor of 45 Second Street, he seemed to me the bravest man in North America. (He didn't really know how to row a boat, and the current was swift and treacherous.) Now, seventy-five years later, the memory of it brings a lump to my throat.

MORCEAUX

I met a first-year medical student at the Lizzie. He writes poems that are quite good, and is dying to be a doctor-poet. Good-looking and clean-cut, he is from a small town in Tennessee. I asked if he knew of Carson-Newman College in Jefferson City, told him that I was being invited there to speak.

"It is a very small, very Southern Baptist school with a great football team." He seemed genuinely surprised that I was being invited.

"Would I be comfortable there?" I asked.

"It would be good for them," he replied. I began to see that the invitation had to do with a piece I wrote long ago, detailing the intra-uterine events of an abortion. It was snatched up by the pro-life crowd, despite that that was contrary to my intention.

"Perhaps," said the student, "you are being sent there for a purpose other than your own." Of course, my appetite has now been whetted. If asked, I will go.

Time was, when I thought of travel as a release, but no more. Now it amounts to carting one old ruin to another one in Rome or Greece or Spain. For me it is not a cure for restlessness but an irritant to that already sensitive skin. I return from wherever I have been not with serenity, appeased, but with greater agitation and frustration than before. Better to let the mind travel while the body stays home.

I used to think of the tree as a lesser creation than the smallest animal that can locomote, while the tree must stay rooted to the spot until it is hewn or toppled. This, to say nothing of the silence of the tree that is devoid of language, incapable of speech. But no more. Against the muteness of the tree is the glossolalia of its leaves. To counteract their immobility, one has only to stand near a maple in the spring and see the little propellers winding downward by the thousand or see a thistle engulfed by an armada of its silken get. Such seedlings can be wafted planetwide by water or wind, or else carried in the entrails of birds, to be deposited far from their parent. No, speak to me not of the silence and immobility of plants; it is animals whose movement and language are the more restricted.

What a strange thing touch is (van Gogh) e.g., the stroke of the brush. There is an electricity about it, a transfer of electrons, of energy. The role of the leader of a workshop is to pose as the model for a painter. To sit still and gaze off to the left.

Letter from a woman who has had a lifelong interest in "striped equids" (zebras). She informed me that no two zebras are exactly alike. Like fingerprints, then.

Happened to be in the room when a newborn baby was handed to its mother. The expression on her face implied that the baby had been sent by Parcel Post rather than delivered otherwise. And from a great distance.

"She stared at the ceiling and hummed a seguidilla through her teeth." Humming is done with the lips; the teeth have nothing to do with it.

All other disappointments pale beside that of the lonely sailor who from the deck of his ship espies a beautiful maiden sitting on a rock in the tide, singing. His heart full of passion, he draws near to listen. He must have her! And tosses his net to capture, only to find that the object of his desire ends in a fish. And not just the tail which might have somehow been gotten around, but the whole bottom half. Here is how Horace put it: "Desinat in piscem mulier formosa superne" (The beautiful damsel ended in a fish).

One antidote for a bad book review is depicted in Swift's "Battle of the Books." It happened that a book had been cut in two by its reviewer. All at once, Venus appeared, took up the severed volume, washed it seven times in ambrosia, and gave it three strokes with a sprig of amaranth. "Upon which, the Leather grew round and soft, the Leaves turned into Feathers, and being gilded before, continued gilded still." So. All one needs is a goddess, a tub of ambrosia, and an amaranth bush.

Interrupted this infernal meandering to give my grandson a bit of instruction in matters of hygiene and deportment. "Having taken a clean handkerchief," I lectured, "you first wipe your glasses, then you blow your nose. Not the other way around." Now that is something useful.

How to Trim an Artichoke

First, prepare yourself as if you were a plastic surgeon about to perform surgery. The poor artichoke is the patient born with any number of congenital deformities that make it unsuitable for acceptance by the other dishes on the table. Let them be veal stew and buttered noodles. What is required is the product of long training, an act of art and craft in equal proportion.

Begin by selecting the sharpest knife and the sturdiest shears in the kitchen cabinet. Now put the artichokes (however many you have) in a deep dishpan full of cold water. Let them soak until most of the brown accumulations have been washed off. Take the first artichoke up in your hand, lay it down on the cutting board, and holding it still with a firm hand, slice off the upper fourth of the fruit. Taking up the shears, insert one blade under the point of each leaf, elevate that part, and cut through. Do this with each leaf. First, you will have broken off the small unusable leaves close to the root. When you have done this, you will amputate the stem leaving one-half of it in situ, as we say in surgery. Using a smaller blade, scrape away any remaining areas of brown discoloration. The artichoke should now be perfectly green and firm. Do this with the other artichokes.

At this point, they must be soaked in a bowl of cold water into which you have squeezed one or two lemons, depending on your lust for lemons. The artichokes can enjoy the cold and cleansing bath for up to an hour. Now transfer them and the lemon water to a steamer. Add sufficient water to cover the grate of the steamer, and place them tightly packed in the standing position into the pan. Cover and heat to boiling, then lower the flame to a slow simmer. After forty minutes, test the ease with which a leaf can be pulled off. Do not test with the point of a knife. If the leaf comes free easily, the artichoke is cooked. It is now perfectly respectable and can be admitted to the dinner table to join its colleagues—veal stew and buttered noodles—without the least hesitation.

Such is the technique of perfecting what nature has left imperfect. Best of all, there is no shedding of blood, and no need to speak to the next of kin waiting in the solarium.

The old house, built in 1912, is moldering. The plumbing gurgles and coughs as in congestive heart failure. Every floorboard has its own distinctive squeak. I don't notice it when Janet is here, but the threadbare carpets, peeling paint, and missing fixtures flaunt themselves in her absence. The mirrors have ceased reflecting. The windowpanes seem to have melted and fused a number of times. The bricks are falling out of the chimneys. We are a mortuary. Only missing is a portrait of myself over the fireplace with my hand on a skull. Number 6 Saint Ronan Terrace is now more like me than I am.

As for conversation at our house, it is sparse. We do not soar above Mumps. Is it singular or plural?

"Plural," she said, but with a bit of uncertainty. "Mumps are . . ." Which gave me no alternative but to say, "Singular . . . Mumps is . . ."

I am like that tiny islet at the far end of an archipelago, the one bypassed by all human life, and abandoned by the gods. Only the occasional migrating bird sets down here to rest before moving on to a real destination. Laughter is not heard here, nor has it happened in several decades. I do not experience joy. The best I can do is reconcile myself to the solitary rummaging in my mind for what to nourish my soul. Oh yes, there are two elderly sheep that go through the motions of grazing among the stones, but there is only a rare blade of grass or a bit of root. Mostly they eat seagrasses that wash up on the beach. Every morning, the ewe comes to stand over my face, and waits for me to open my eyes. She bleats once or twice until I reach up and press the thin milk from her nipple into my throat. Unfortunately, it is enough to keep me alive.

As the sole occupant of the islet, I am both its king and its subject. As such I have given myself the gift of dreaming. One dream that occurs with some frequency is that the islet comes unmoored from its attachments to the sea bottom and floats off in search of a continent to which it might become attached by a narrow isthmus across which a wanderer might find his way. One day, it happened just in this way. A family of three—mother, father, and infant son—appeared at this end of the isthmus. How the sheep stared at them! In keeping with my kingly presence, I held my excitement in check and strolled down to bid them welcome.

"What is the child's name?" I asked.

"Rhapsody," said the mother. Just then, a great eagle flew low over our heads, and a rainbow appeared in the eastern sky transforming this dessicated speck of land into something Persian.

In book 6 of the *Aeneid*, Aeneas has met up with his father, Anchises, in the Elysian Fields. They come upon a crowd of souls waiting by a river. Anchises explains that they are awaiting the summons to new bodies, and must drink of the waters of the river Lethe in order to learn forgetfulness of their past lives. Sometimes, mostly at noon and at midnight, those two hinges of the day, I have the fleeting memory that my own father had once conducted me just as Anchises had led Aeneas, that he had bade me join those who were destined to come back, only, for some reason—disobedience, I suppose—I didn't drink of the waters of forgetfulness, and so it is that I know full well what I had been in a former life—a surgeon.

It was from my father's medical textbooks that I first encountered the language of medicine. *Arteriosclerosis*, I read, and thought it sounded like a ruby that is worn about the neck. And *carcinoma*, which sounded like *cara nome*, that aria from *Rigoletto* that my mother used to sing . . . I was never seen without the elderly, tattered doctor's bag that followed me about on my rounds for thirty years. It was far more learned than I ever was—fluent in Hebrew, Latin, French, and Algebra, it understood Archimedes' principle. It was a descendant of my father's black doctor's bag that, all by itself, could perform an appendectomy, or so he swore.

A Parable

The scene is a room at the hospital. I am standing in the open doorway. It is early morning. A man is lying in the bed. He is emaciated, his skin covered with purple blotches where the blood has leaked into the tissues and congealed. He is motionless, inert. Only his breathing gives evidence of life. It comes in short, rapid bursts interrupted by long stretches of apnea, as though a creature sat astride him and rode him till he could not take a breath. Then it would start in again. It is called Cheyne-Stokes respiration. When the patient starts that, you know it won't be long. There is suppuration around his eyes, blocking his vision. He makes no effort to clear the phlegm rattling in his throat, only coughs mechanically now and then. It is clear that he is dying.

A doctor, at least I presume he is a doctor, comes into the room. I step aside to let him pass. He is wearing a blue scrub suit such as is worn in the operating theater. He is elderly, with hair the color of pewter and blue eyes. His arms are thin and hairless and white. They end in hands that seem too large and heavy for the arms. They are red and shiny from years of scrubbing with stiff brushes. He takes a tissue, moistens it and wipes the purulence from the sick man's eyes, which I can now see are dark, the color of wet stones. They move to bring the doctor into focus. From the doorway of the room where I am standing, I see the lips of the doctor move, but I cannot hear what he is saying. He bends closer, placing his mouth almost to the man's ear, and raises his voice. Now what I hear is a soft humming. During the night the patient has slid down in the bed and has gotten knotted among the sheets. The doctor slides one hand beneath the patient's hips and the other beneath his shoulders and lifts him up, embracing him, enclosing him as if his arms were a cloak or a hiding place where the man in his misery might rest safe and secure.

The man in the bed tries to speak, but his voice is broken, fissured, bleeding, and he cannot. All that emerges are syllables in their larval state, mangled, and coagulated in a viscous unintelligible soup. From where I stand, I imagine that the sick body is hot, so hot that it gives forth warmth, like a rock that has lain out in the sun. A steam seems to rise from the bed. The old doctor holds his hands over the body of the man as if to warm them. The man makes another effort to speak. When the doctor turns his head to bend an ear to the lips of his patient, I can see the deep furrow that divides his brow, extending from the bridge of the nose up almost to the hairline. It is a line of pain. Had he been born with it, I wonder. No, I think he had not. Rather, it had appeared on the day that he treated his first patient. At first it was merely a shadow on his forehead, then a slight indentation that over the years has deepened into this dark cleft that is the mark of all the suffering he has witnessed over a lifetime as a doctor. It resembles a wound that might have been made with an ax.

Now the doctor lowers his hands into the heat and the steam and places them on the naked abdomen. Gently he presses, palpating, all the while speaking.

"Am I hurting you?" he asks—or is it the hands themselves that ask the question? The man in the bed shakes his head. All at once (who would have thought he had the strength?) he raises one trembling hand and moves it toward the doctor's head. Could it be that the doctor bends forward a little so as to bring his cloven brow within reach? The sick man finds the furrow with his finger, touches, then strokes it from one end to the other, a look of wonder on his face, as though he were just waking from a deep sleep. As he does so, a spicule of light appears to emanate from the doctor's forehead. It is a warm light that grows to engulf the two men and the bed. From this touching, the doctor does not withdraw, but smiles down at the patient with his sapphiric gaze.

The doctor covers the man's abdomen and lifts the sheet to expose his feet. They are blue and, I think, cold despite the fever. The doctor takes one foot in his hand and begins to massage it gently, the way you rub the blood into a frozen part of the body. The man closes his eyes as if to concentrate the comfort he feels. His breathing slows and eases. Within minutes, he is asleep.

From the doorway, the two men and the bed appear luminous. They exist in a miraculous light. Miraculous? Why not? There are certain moments of harmony and revelation when miracles might be expected. They seem right and proper, like the luminous glow that has appeared to envelop the sick man and his doctor so that they themselves seem to be composed of light. Indeed, if there had been no miraculous light about them, it would have been astonishing.

It is as if I were witnessing a feast. As if a table has been set with linen and plates and silverware. Candles have been lit. Ah, so that is the source of the light! There is bread in a small basket, and wine in the goblets. The two men are dining together, each the nourishment of the other.

Bit of conversation with a student:

> HE: How are you?
> ME: Old and scrawny.
> HE: You said that the last time I asked you.
> ME: Well there you are. I'm old, scrawny, and repetitive.

There's a certain Slant of light
Winter Afternoons—
That oppresses, like the Heft
Of Cathedral Tunes—

. . . .

When it comes, the Landscape listens—
Shadows—hold their breath—
When it goes, 'tis like the Distance
On the look of Death—

Emily Dickinson

Ran into Henri Peyre, esteemed professor of French, at the card catalogue. He was looking in the P's. He told me that he needs a new prostate.
I said I doubted he would find one in the card catalogue.

"Nobody needs me anymore." He gave a Gallic shrug. "Why should
I write?"

"Think of Montaigne," I advised. "He had a prostate too."

"Ah yes, Montaigne, he had to make peepee all the time. He had
stones. At least I don't have stones, not yet. Old age . . ." He rolled his
eyes, giving the words all the passion of Phèdre attacked by the talons of
Venus. ("Ce n'est plus un ardeur dans mes veines caché; c'est Vénus toute
entière a sa proie attaché." Or something like that.)

"You should read him again," I suggested.

"Who?"

"Montaigne—his essay on how to die."

"My God! I am not that bad yet!"

Donating one's body for dissection in an anatomy laboratory is more than just carrying one's funeral pyre around with him; it is a triumph over death, a way of realizing immortality. Once the knowledge has been imparted to the fledgling doctors, what is left is cremated for the sake of cleanliness and hygiene.

The King, Hamlet's father, died "unhousled," with all his sins upon his head, and impenitent. That is how I shall go, I'm afraid, trusting upon divine leniency to accept me with all my imperfections.

Two noisily dressed students at the Beinecke Library. One, a girl in a taffeta skirt. The crepitus! The hissing! And at the next table, a fat boy in corduroy pants. Whenever his thighs rubbed together, there came that metallic whine. At the first sound of either, the Muse took cover. Were I in charge, I'd excommunicate both taffeta and corduroy from the libraries of America. And the students insist on conversing aloud in the library. In my next life, I am going to be a silentiary, not in a Trappisarium but in a library. My chief duty would be to shush.

ON WRITING

I no longer teach anatomy to medical students; I lead workshops for them in creative writing. (I never thought I'd sink so low.)

To become a writer, you must activate the third eye, the one that sits in between the eyebrows and is covered over with skin. This is best done by long periods of daydreaming. After a while, you will feel, in the middle of the forehead, a slight itching that no amount of scratching will relieve. In time this itching will grow into a feeling of pressure, as though something living were trapped thereunder. Something is. Surgery is of no use except in the famous case of Dr. Hua Po in ancient China. One day a man visited Hua Po complaining of a terrible itching between the eyes. Examination revealed a swelling there. When Hua Po took up his knife and cut open the swelling, out flew a canary, which sat on the man's shoulder and sang all day long. (But I digress.)

Soon you will notice that the skin of your forehead has begun to flake. Strange wrinkles appear. At last, there is a sudden ripping sensation, followed by a blinding light. Immediately the pressure vanishes, and there it is, the third eye, open and unblinking and seeing what no one else can, the glowing center of things. All right, now you are a writer, but you are also a monstrosity whose appearance is upsetting to your friends. They will shun you. "Here comes Old Three-Eyes," they'll say and cross themselves or spit over a shoulder. Most likely, they will try to cover your third eye with their hand so that you will not perceive them as they really are. Poor things! They don't know that your eye can see through everything.

If given the choice between teaching anatomy or creative writing, I'd go fishing.

❧

My own best writing has been in the medical charts of my patients. It is the only writing of mine that is free of the pomp of language and the vanity of the author. It is also writing that had great importance to the patient and his doctor, to both of whom it was a matter of life and death. In some as yet unrealized way it is related to my decision to donate my body to the Medical School for anatomical dissection by the students. It is a way of living on after death, of continuing to be useful, and it beats the heck out of being buried in the ground beneath a carved stone.

❧

I read somewhere that Madame Jeanne Roland, condemned to death by the Revolutionary Tribunal in 1793, asked at the foot of the guillotine for pen and paper, which were denied her. Unlike Madame Roland, I carry pen and notebook with me wherever I go, just in case I am surprised by a worthy metaphor. Having had to write catch-as-catch-can while practicing surgery—in fifteen minute bursts—I can write anywhere, anytime. That is unlike Rilke, say, who had to live in isolated castles with all the furniture arranged just so. I carry my imagination in a bandanna tied to a stick. That way, I can take it out and give it an airing any time I want.

I am well aware of the sexual ambiguity that is openly revealed in the characters of my stories. Many of the males are attracted to other men in loving friendship that veers close to the physical. As in Walt Whitman's wound-dresser, the body of a wounded soldier is cherished by the male nurse. Sometimes, in the throes of writing, I feel that I have a woman's soul that has somehow gotten displaced into the body of a man. Far from being ashamed of what others might call perversion or imposture, I credit it with a good deal of my literary creativity. The essence of good doctoring is the acceptance of the sick and wounded as having no rigid gender but as human beings with the virtues and faults of both male and female.

Some things are beyond words. Only music, painting, or sculpture can come close to realizing them. Language falls short (Shakespeare's excepted). The writer has the impossible task of moving the Pillars of Hercules one millimeter during his lifetime. Of course, it can't be done. Instead he has to titrate passion and nonexistence drop by drop until the litmus tells him that the precise pH of art has been reached. Painting and sculpture, unlike writing, are silent, voiceless. They converse by pathways other than words. Their message and its response are swift and powerful. Language, on the other hand, must be read and argued.

There are those who will tell you that a narrative should be as straight and flexible as a clothesline with socks and underwear hanging out to dry. But my writings are all knotted and twisted to conform to the gyri and sulci of this damaged article, my brain, which is incapable of organized thought anymore, and is only subject to purposeless eddies of the blood.

To describe a still life, try to relate physics to metaphysics. Go from the objects themselves through thought and emotion to mystery. The effect that the objects have upon one another, and the effect of light and shadow on the objects.

❧

Like Schopenhauer, I am depressed by thoughts of the Australian bulldog ant. Cut this creature in half, and it fights with itself, head against tail. Head seizes tail in its teeth, tail stings head, back and forth until one or both are dead. How can one hope for peace on earth when violence is inherent in the act of living? It is instinctive. In writing, act instinctively. Without cogitation. Instinct cannot be understood, only obeyed blindly. It is inexplicable, as in the savagery of the bisected bulldog ant.

❧

There is the matter of tone, which can be high as in *Wuthering Heights*, low, as in *Huckleberry Finn*, or middling as in the works of all those who can't sustain a high or low tone throughout the course of a book. Tone establishes the relationship between reader and writer. If Eve had been tempted by a turnip instead of an apple, the book of Genesis would have had a lower tone. It would deserve the term "Vulgate."

As Lady Margaret Beaumont said at dinner next to Henry Adams, "I don't think I care for foreigners," an example of the application of high tone to low character.

It is twenty-five years since first I wet a pen, and nobody can say I have been a *lazzarone*. Or, I've been writing for twenty-five years, and you can't say I've loafed.

⊱⊰

The worst sin of a doctor is arrogance, the conviction that he is right and beyond questioning. Many a patient has suffered unnecessary and contra-indicated treatment on the advice of arrogant doctors. But such is not the case in storytelling, where both reader and writer are insulated from personal injury by the transfer of reality to the pages of a book.

I confess that I have a good deal of trouble understanding modern poetry. So much of it seems to have been made purposely obscure. One argument in favor of such obscurity is that a wild bird doesn't permit itself to be seen readily, and so it engages in all sorts of disguises in order to fool the birdwatcher. But at age eighty, I haven't time for such a game. I'd better make it all clear now.

There is also, in this hard-bitten age, the sense that sentimentality is to be avoided by the storyteller at all times. I would take a different tack. To be sentimental is to take pleasure in humble things—filial devotion, natural beauty, the overcoming of great odds. I think of the poem "Trees" by Joyce Kilmer, once required to be recited by every fifth-grade student in North America:

> I think that I shall never see
> A poem lovely as a tree.
>
> A tree whose hungry mouth is prest
> Against the earth's sweet flowing breast;
>
> A tree that looks at God all day,
> And lifts her leafy arms to pray;

A tree that may in summer wear
A nest of robins in her hair;

Upon whose bosom snow has lain;
Who intimately lives with rain.

Poems are made by fools like me,
But only God can make a tree.

Even an old skeptic such as I can respond to the religious impulse that
drives the poet.

It is four days since the staged readings of the play adapted from my story
"Diary of an Infidel" were presented, and I am trying to decide what
made the utterance of the piece so much more moving and powerful than
the text on a page. The written piece is akin to death, while the staged
reading has a living immediacy. Through the voice of the actors, "Infidel"
rose out of bloodless inertia and became living speech. If it were given to
me, I would cross over from writing into speech or song. It is precisely
that which makes the operas of Verdi so much more powerful than their
plots. In the matter of illness, such as the abbot's carbuncle, it can never be
fully portrayed in written words no matter the fluency of the writer.
There is always something that remains mysterious, secret, undisclosed—
the true suffering of the sick and the wounded. Only the living outcry of
pain from the abbot himself could deliver it. That is what literature
attempts to do, but it is an impossible quest.

One symptom of old age is the inability to control one's emotions. I
confess to having shed tears while reading my story "Atrium" aloud

before an audience of residents in internal medicine. If this be thought egotism, at least it testifies to the sincerity with which the story was created. It is the opposite of Dante's passage through the dark wood in his descent into Hell.

In the story the boy goes willingly to his death under the tutelage of the doctor. The release of his body into Nature is rendered in ceremonial terms. It is a rite of passage conducted in a world other than the strictly human. The doctor crosses a line in order to achieve the transfer of the boy from his mortality into Nature. I think of Priam, king of Troy, who crossed another line in order to retrieve the body of his son Hector from Achilles, the Greek warrior who slew him. The aged Priam enters the camp of the Greeks accompanied by Hermes, the messenger of the gods. When Achilles and Priam meet, they see each other as fellow sufferers. Priam kneels and kisses the hands of Achilles. Achilles' heart melts and he agrees to give the body of Hector to his father. Life can go on. But unlike Priam, the doctor in "Atrium" is not granted repose. He is haunted by the image of the boy lying in the shadowy forest. Dramatic art arises from the dilemmas and mysteries of life; it makes no promise to relieve or solve anything. Still, the further this real event retreats into time past, the subtler the effect of the story, until it touches, like the pressure of a sunbeam. With time, it takes on the color of myth or fairy tale.

Each story or essay I write changes the shape of my mind, so that the next story or essay will be written by someone else, someone a little different from the man I used to be. I imagine the same is true of a great actor. Every role he plays becomes incorporated for better or worse into his personality. That cannot be said about a craftsman who does the same thing over and over.

There are certain things you should know about a writer. A writer is desperate and merciless. His sole wish is to take words prisoner and hold them captive without hope of escape. He is at the same time a child rummaging in the closet of a grownup, forever trying on different clothes. Like most storytellers, I have a certain amount of contempt for the facts. I prefer impressions. Impressions are what last; they're more reliable than facts. Impressions are often what determine the course of our lives; love at first sight, for instance. Facts have a tendency to change every generation or so. Facts are devoid of morality and romance. To Hell with facts! In a story entitled "Pages from a Wound-Dresser's Diary," when it came time for a hospital steamboat, the *January,* to hide from a Rebel "ram"—a boat equipped with a pointed steel prow for ramming into enemy ships—I looked on a map of the South for the name of a river under whose vines and creepers I could have my *January* conceal itself. I found just such a river, called the Yazoo. And so it happened in my story. No sooner had this piece been published in a magazine than the wrath and scorn of a multitude of Civil War buffs fell upon me. The mail was voluminous and vituperative. Didn't I know that in 1863 the Yazoo River had not yet been dredged and could have hidden nothing larger than a rowboat? Well, no, I didn't. When the time came to include the story in a book, I had the chance to correct the gaffe, to choose another river. Did I? Of course not. I had fallen in love with the name Yazoo, and no contemptible insistence upon the facts could cause me to be untrue.

Suturing, either with a pen and ink or needle and thread, produces something that is born of the imagination of the creator. Whether of cloth or language, it has been touched by the gentle treason of art. The unicorn embroidered on a pillowcase is no less remarkable than the unicorn portrayed in words on a page, and it is just as strong a stimulus to the dreams of the child whose head rests upon it. I suspect that the song of such a "pillowed" bird is more accessible to the ear of a dreamer than the song of a bird trapped in a cage of words.

In order to write, it is not necessary to lead a quiet, peaceful life. On the contrary, conflict and misery are often the stimuli for creative writing.

What is now this book (*Knife Song Korea*) was written first as a journal of my stay in Korea. Somewhere along the way, I felt it necessary to turn it into fictional form. By the time I returned to surgery at Yale, I had repressed the writing of the novel. It simply did not exist until January 2007, some twenty years after my retirement from surgery. In the intervening years I had embarked on what was to become a second career, that of a writer. It happened that the Institute of the Medical Humanities took an interest in my work and provided the funds for the acquisition of my papers by the library of the University of Texas Medical Branch in Galveston. It was a great relief to gather up the piles and piles of paper and ship it all to Texas unsorted and unexamined. Unbeknownst to me, the manuscript of the Korean story was among those papers. In January 2007, more than fifty years after it was written, I received a phone call from a scholar who, rummaging in the Archive, came upon this story.

"I've just read your novel," he said.

"There must be some mistake," I replied. "I have never written a novel."

"But," he persisted, "I have it in my hand, even as we speak."

"What's the name of it?" I asked.

" 'The Bronze Gong,' " he told me. "Look here, I'll have it copied and send it to you."

Before I could persuade him not to do that, there it was in my mailbox. A manuscript titled "The Bronze Gong," by Richard Selzer.

Imagine the trepidation I felt as I began to read for the first time what I had written more than half a century earlier, long before I became Richard Selzer, writer. It is a story conceived and executed in utero, as it were. Right from the first page, the whole of that Korean experience came tumbling back in all its horror and violence and tragedy. For fifty-three years, the manuscript had lain in hibernation. Now, it has been "tidied up" and undergone a change in title. As *Knife Song Korea* it has been resurrected. What do I think of it? There is a certain freshness, a lack of sophistication, as well as an absence of the vanity of the author and the pomp of language that some of my later works have. Beyond that, I cannot say.

As far as my own biography is concerned, it is a kind of fool's errand. I haven't really lived. I've tried to dissuade the woman who is determined to do it; she is wasting her time. But it is hard to quench a heart on fire. I can only hope that she has not somehow found me out—I should hate for my children to discover that their father is more to be censured than pitied. If anyone should ask me how I live my life, I say that I sit in a deep chair all day and I read. It is a way of avoiding responsibility, of avoiding life. That is no fit subject for a biography.

I read in the biography of William Butler Yeats that the Spanish doctor who attended the poet on Majorca reported to his Irish colleague, "We have here an antique cardiosclerotic of advanced years." When he returned to Ireland, Yeats asked his doctor to read the report aloud.

"Read it slowly and distinctly," he ordered, then inclined his head, following the cadence with his finger. As the sound died away, Yeats exclaimed, "Do you know, I would rather be called an antique cardiosclerotic than Lord of Lower Egypt."

crat 8/11
OK 9/11
TAP 11/12
CG 3/14
OK 8/14
SGR 7/15
OK 6/16
BAN 7/16
CG 3/18